Nanoparticles in Humans

Nanoparticles in Humans

Experiments, Methods, and Strategies

Lev S. Ruzer

Pan Stanford Publishing

Published by

Pan Stanford Publishing Pte. Ltd.
Penthouse Level, Suntec Tower 3
8 Temasek Boulevard
Singapore 038988

Email: editorial@panstanford.com
Web: www.panstanford.com

British Library Cataloguing-in-Publication Data
A catalogue record for this book is available from the British Library.

Nanoparticles in Humans: Experiments, Methods, and Strategies

ISBN 978-981-4463-16-4 (Hardcover)
ISBN 978-981-4463-17-1 (eBook)

FSC
www.fsc.org
MIX
Paper from responsible sources
FSC® C013056

Printed and bound in Great Britain by
TJ International Ltd, Padstow, Cornwall

I dedicate this work to my dearest friend,
Professor Tatjana Tolstikova

Contents

Preface

The history of radon and the associated health effect (lung cancer) is very long—from the 15th century—and it consists of two parts: radon in mines and residential radon. In the majority of studies, radon measurements were provided as a proof of the effect (lung cancer). However, radon is an inert gas, and it is not precipitated (not remained) in the lung. Therefore, it cannot be completely responsible for lung irradiation and correspondingly lung cancer. Radon progeny precipitate in the lung. They also can precipitate to the particles, including particles in the nanometer range, and therefore they can be used as radioactive markers in the study of nanoparticles.

This book presents new ideas, methods, and some experimental results to measure the surface area and local deposition of nanoparticles in lungs and the true effectiveness of respirators, together with a nanoparticle dosimetric road map that can be used as a general strategy for the assessment of dose, which is the most important physical cause of the health effect in case of nanoparticle exposure. It proposes the use of 1 nm radioactive particles, called unattached activity of radon progeny, as a safe experimental tool for nanoparticle studies, including human studies. Such ideas have not been presented before. The text includes some discussion on radon from the historical point of view.

Acknowledgments

I appreciate the support of the Environmental Energy Technology Division of Lawrence Berkeley National Laboratory and thank William Fisk, Ashok Gadgil, Olivia Salazar, and Terry Chen for the technical help. I am also grateful to my family—my son, Serge Ruzer; my daughter, Genia, and her husband, Sasha; and especially my grandchildren, Joseph, Liza, Ada, and Simona—for their variegated technical assistance.

Chapter 1

Radon Deadlock

We are not rich enough to buy cheap things.
—Proverb

1.1 Radon and Health

The history of health problems associated with radon goes back to the towns of Schneeberg and Jachymov, where mining started in the early 15th century (Lewis, 2006).

Mining in those very early years was done for silver, copper, and iron and later for cobalt- and arsenic-containing ores. After the discovery of uranium, it was found that the ore contained about 1% uranium. Uranium, at that time, was used for coloring wood, leather, pottery glazes, and glass.

The conditions in mines were very poor. According to Agricola, "the dust has corrosive qualities, it eats away the lungs and implants consumption in the body... Women are found who have married seven husbands, all of whom this terrible consumption has carried off to a premature death." The miners themselves called this disease "bergsucht" or "mountain sickness."

Nanoparticles in Humans: Experiments, Methods, and Strategies
Lev S. Ruzer

ISBN 978-981-4463-16-4 (Hardcover), 978-981-4463-17-1 (eBook)
www.panstanford.com

The cause of the problem was only later understood after the discovery of x-rays in 1895 by W. C. Roentgen, radioactivity in 1896 by Henri Becquerel, radium in 1898 by M. Curie and P. Curie, and finally radon by Friedrich Ernst Dorn in 1900, initially called "radium emanation"—it was not called radon until 1923.

In 1879, Harting and Hesse proved that the "mountain sickness" among the Schneeberg miners was actually a malignant tumor of the lung. They showed that from 1869 to 1877 about, 75% of deaths among the miners of Schneeberg were due to lung cancer.

At that time, the calculated dose of radon to the lung was too small to produce the effects seen in comparison with radium doses and external radiation doses associated with carcinogenesis. The answer to this problem will be obvious to most of researchers. The decay scheme for radium had already been worked out and people knew that there were "daughters." However, few researchers made measurements to characterize the decay products. In 1944, Lorenz even pointed out that radon contributed only a few percent of the dose from an equilibrium mixture. In the early 1950s, Dr. John Harley (1953) may also be given credit for his identical ideas in his PhD work. Thus, it is really the radon decay products that deliver the significant dose to the lungs, far more so than the radon gas.

This fact had been overlooked in all past studies.

The special role of radon progeny was underlined in papers and books by this author. Even in the first paper published on this subject (Ruzer, 1958), the quantities' assessment—both theoretically and experimentally—was presented. That paper and others on comparative contribution to the dose and health effect of radon and radon progeny were published in the Soviet journal *Atomnaya Energiya* (in Russian). The complete study for radon and its progeny, including animal and human (miners) measurements and epidemiology (lung cancer sickness and mortality), was later presented in Ruzer (2001) (in Russian), and Ruzer (2012), and Ruzer et al. (2004).

News had spread quickly from Europe to the United States regarding the discovery and uses of radium and uranium. Beginning in the late 1890s, exploration and mining began in Utah, Colorado, Arizona, and New Mexico. During these early years, uranium was mined for the extraction of radium. In fact, much of this uranium was shipped to Pennsylvania for radium production from 1912 to 1920. Radium was thought to be a new wonder substance for the treatment of many maladies. Uranium was still being used as a coloring agent in glass, and vanadium, often found with uranium, was used to harden steel. This mining continued until the 1940s. The Manhattan Project caused a shift in what uranium was used for. In 1948, uranium was the ultimate goal of the production of uranium-235 and plutonium.

The residential history of radon—and associated national health risk-related issues—started in 1984, when it was found that the home of an engineer, working at the nuclear plant in Pennsylvania, had an exceptionally high concentration of radon in the basement, close to 2,700 Pico curies per L, which is more than an order of magnitude higher than most miners are exposed to. The resulting media attention led to radon's being labeled a major public health problem.

From 1986 to the present, many studies have been conducted on radon and radon-associated health effects. However, in the majority of the studies until now, radon itself, not radon progeny, was measured as a cause of lung cancer. However, radon is an inert gas. It not precipitated in the lung. Therefore, it cannot substantially irradiate the lung and cannot be considered a direct cause of lung cancer (Ruzer, 2012).

As a result, we have now a situation described in *JCEN* (2011): "The handling of radon as a public health risk by Environment Protection Agency USA over the past 25 years has been long on talk but short on results."

We illustrate this with the results of two studies: BEIR VI and Darby et al. (2004). It should be mentioned that in BEIR VI a great work was accomplished: The distribution of radon and its progeny concentrations in mines of 11 different countries were presented and analyzed together with data on lung cancer mortality among miners.

In Darby, et al., the similar very important data on radon were presented. Again, the authors did a very good job in collecting and analyzing information on the distribution of radon concentration in Europe. Unfortunately, they try to connect radon concentration

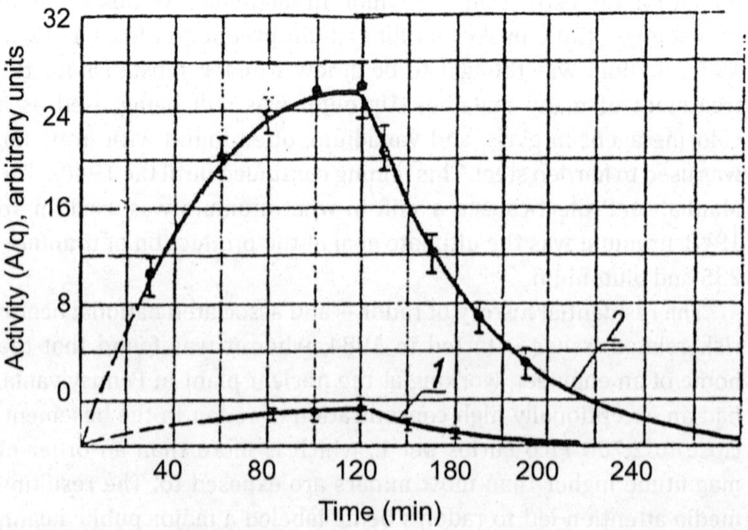

Figure 1.1 Buildup and clearance of radon (1) and buildup and decay of radon progeny (2) in rats. Copyright (2012). From *Aerosols Handbook: Measurement, Dosimetry, and Health Effects*, Second Edition, edited by Lev S. Ruzer and Naomi H. Harley. Reproduced by permission of Taylor and Francis Group, LLC, a division of Informa plc.

itself with lung cancer mortality of the general population despite the fact that only radon progeny, not radon itself, is responsible for the biological effect. So, it is a classic case when not a dose as a cause of the effect, but rather the dose's surrogate was studied, and the correlation and the real cause were not established. But that is not all.

In Table D-12 of BEIR VI, results of average exposures in working levels (WLM) are presented for 11 countries (China 286.0, Czechoslovakia 196.8, France 59.4, Canada and USA 578.6, etc.). We know that the uncertainty in the exposure assessment is in the order at least of tens of percent. Therefore, we cannot trust these data with tenths of WLMs.

Our study on dosimetry and health effect on miners in Tajikistan (Ruzer et al., 1995) suggested that different groups of miners got substantially different exposure (dose) and different lung

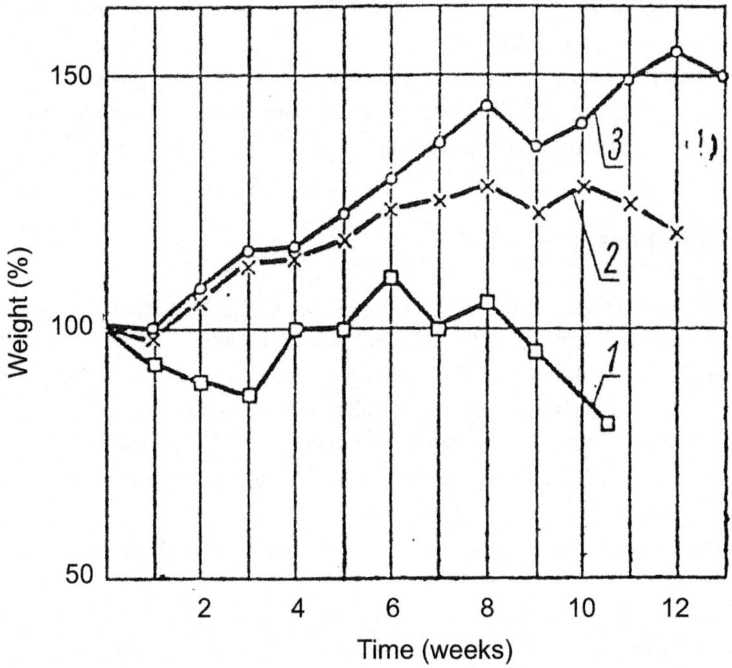

Figure 1.2 Weight of animals exposed to radon: (1) First series; (2) second series; (3) third series and control. Copyright (2012). From *Aerosols Handbook: Measurement, Dosimetry, and Health Effects*, Second Edition, edited by Lev S. Ruzer and Naomi H. Harley. Reproduced by permission of Taylor and Francis Group, LLC, a division of Informa plc.

cancer mortality. So averaging in this case can lead to additional uncertainty.

It seems that in some of epidemiological studies, there exists a tendency to present as much as possible cases of effect (mortality, morbidity, etc.) in order to get good statistics. With such tendency, we often use old and questionable data on concentrations, even based on data on ventilation. Therefore, our good statistics on mortality in such cases are compromised with bad dosimetry.

As shown in Ruzer (2012), for correct assessment of relative contribution of radon itself and its progeny, it is necessary to measure separately the activity of radon and its decay products *in the body, not only in the air,* as it was done in experiments on animals (see Figs. 1.1 and 1.2).

In the following chapters, we will describe the properties of radon progeny, including those which can be used as a marker in the study of nanometer particles.

References

BEIR VI (1999) *Health Effect of Exposure to Radon*, National Research Council, Washington, DC, National Academy Press.

Darby S, Hill D, Auvinen A, BarrosDios JM, Baysson H, et al. (2004) Radon in homes and risk of lung cancer: Collaborative analysis of individual data from 13 European case-control studies. *BMJ* **330**(7485), 223.

Harley JH (1953) Sampling and measurement of airborne daughter products of radon. *Nucleonics*, **11**, July 12–15.

Journal Chemical and Engineering News (JCEN), American Chemical Society, August 22, 2011.

Lewis RK (2006) *A History of Radon: 1470 to 1984*, Presented at the 2006 National Radon Meeting, 2006. http://www.ohioradonpro.com.

Ruzer LS (1958) *Atomnaya Energiya*, 189–194, February.

Ruzer LS (2001) *Radioactive Aerosols*, Energoizdat, Moscow, Russia.

Ruzer LS (2012) Radon deadlock, *ANRI*, #2 (69), 62–66 (in Russian).

Ruzer LS, Harley NH (2005) *Aerosol Handbook: Measurement, Dosimetry, and Health Effects*. New York, CRC Press.

Ruzer LS, Harley NH (2005) *Aerosol Handbook: Measurement, Dosimetry, and Health Effects*, 2nd ed. New York, CRC Press.

Ruzer, LS, Nero, AV, Harley, NH (1995) Assessment of lung deposition and breathing rate of underground miners in Tadjikistan. *Radiation Prot Dosimetry*, **58**, 261–265.

Chapter 2

Measurement of the Concentration of Decay Products of Radon, Thoron, and Actinon

2.1 Characteristics of Radon Progeny

The presence of radon and its decay products is due to the abundance in the earth of heavy metals—radioactive elements at the end of the periodic table. One of them, uranium, undergoes a long series of transformations to yield radium. The chain of radioactive decay does continue further; however, nature dictates that the member of the chain after radium, radon, is a radioactive noble gas. Owing to its inert chemical properties, radon does not remain in the earth or in water but enters the atmosphere. The links that follow in the radioactive chain—isotopes of polonium, bismuth, and lead—attach to aerosol particles to become radioactive aerosols or exist in the unattached form in the air. Eventually, they may be deposited in the lungs and cause irradiation to the lung tissue.

Specific biological consequences depend on the amount (concentration) of radioactive aerosols and also on the physiological characteristics of human beings, especially physical activity. The concentration depends not only on the amount of the radium in the

Nanoparticles in Humans: Experiments, Methods, and Strategies
Lev S. Ruzer

ISBN 978-981-4463-16-4 (Hardcover), 978-981-4463-17-1 (eBook)
www.panstanford.com

soil and in the air but also on atmospheric conditions in the open air, dwellings, and underground environment.

The greatest health concern is from alpha emitters, because the alpha particles have the greatest ionization density (Linear Energy Transfer [LET]). Given identical absorbed energy, the biological effect of alpha particles is supposed to be 20 times greater than the corresponding effect of beta particles and gamma radiation (the "quality coefficient" for alpha particles is 20).

However, it is practically impossible to measure the alpha activity of aerosols deposited in the lungs of a living subject. As a result, this alpha radioactivity should be measured in the air, and the absorbed dose to the lungs is then calculated according to the known concentration, breathing rate, and the coefficient of deposition in the lungs. The concentration of radon in the open air depends to a large extent on atmospheric conditions and on the air movement.

The average concentration of radon decay products in the atmosphere fluctuates between 4 and 40 Bq/m^3. However, there are instances when local or temporary concentrations are two orders of magnitudes higher. In closed premises, whether buildings, residences, or mines, the concentration depends much on the rate of ventilation as it does on the amount of radon in the soil (construction materials) and in water.

The measurement of the concentration of the natural radioactive aerosol—decay products of radon, thoron, and actinon—is important not only due to its own irradiation of the lungs. With the advent of nuclear power and nuclear weapons systems, artificial radioactive aerosols began to enter the air because of nuclear experiments, leakages of radioactive substances, and nuclear accidents. In this sense, it should be pointed out that the background natural radioactive aerosols are serious obstacle to the correct measurement of artificial radioactive aerosol concentration.

It should be pointed out that the maximum permissible concentration (MPC) for artificial radioactive aerosols, especially for alpha emitters, are two to three orders of magnitudes lower than the concentrations of radon decay products in the atmosphere.

Thus, in measuring the concentration of artificial radioactive aerosols, which are mostly long-lived isotopes, two different approaches can be used:

1. Using "waiting method," i.e., make the measurements only after the short-lived decay products of radon and thoron will decay substantially enough (sometimes for 3–4 days after sampling); such an approach is not always acceptable in practical situations.
2. Using spectroscopic methods. Even with this type of technique, the natural radioactive aerosol background together with aerosol concentration itself will play a substantial role and should be taken into account.

2.2 The Basic Equations for Radon Decay Product Series

The basic equations in the most generalized form for the radon series were derived in Ruzer (1958) and Ruzer (1968). The derivations were based on the equations described in Bateman (1910) with some transformations. For the determination of the correlation between the measured concentration and activity of each decay product on the filter, the Bateman equation for the chain of radioactive transformations was used.

To insert these equations into the mechanism of the buildup activity on the filter due to filtration (or physiological breathing), we assumed that the first member of this chain for each decay product are the decay products in the air, which supply the decay products to the lungs with a constant rate $Q_i = q_i vk/\lambda_i$.

From the mathematical point of view, the constant rate of supply is equal to the equilibrium between the first and the second member of the chain of radioactive transformation. In this case, the number of the atoms, N, of each decay products in the lungs can be found according to the following equation:

$$N_i = c_1 e^{-\lambda_1 t} + c_2 e^{-\lambda_2 t} + \cdots + c_i e^{-\lambda_i t}, \tag{2.1}$$

where

$$c_i = N_{1,0} \cdot \lambda_1 \lambda_1 \lambda_2 \ldots \lambda_{i-1} / (\lambda_1 - \lambda_i)(\lambda_2 - \lambda_i) \ldots (\lambda_{i-1} - \lambda_i). \tag{2.2}$$

Let us examine the quantitative correlation between the activity $A_i(\theta, t)$ of a given isotope on a filter, correspondently to a given duration of filtration (breathing) θ, time after the conclusion of filtration (exposure) t, and concentration of each decay products q_i. We will assume first that the concentrations for the duration of filtration do not change, the radioactivity on the filter is affected only by the short-lived radon decay products, and the coefficients of retention are identical for each decay product.

It is also presupposed that during the time of the sampling, the basic parameters of the aerosol system are constant.

The Activity of ^{214}Bi (RaC) on the filter $A_c(\theta, t)$ is made up of ^{214}Bi (RaC), which has deposited during filtration taking into account its decay $A_{c,c}(\theta, t)$ and also of ^{214}Bi (RaC) formed as result of the decay of ^{218}Po (RaA) – $A_{c,a}(\theta, t)$ and of ^{214}Pb (RaB) – $A_{c,b}(\theta, t)$.

The formulas for each of these activities can be obtained by applying Eqs. (2.1) and (2.2). We will provide the equations in two steps. First, Eqs. (2.1) and (2.2) will be used for describing the changes taking place on the filter after sampling. At the moment t after completion of the sample activity is

$$A_{c,a}(\theta, t) = A_a(\theta, 0)\lambda_b\lambda_c.\{[(e^{-\lambda_b^t} - e^{-\lambda_a^t})/(\lambda_a - \lambda_b)(\lambda_c - \lambda_c b)] + [(e^{-\lambda_c^t} - e^{-\lambda_a^t})/(\lambda_a - \lambda_c)(\lambda_b - \lambda_c)]\}; \quad (2.3)$$

$$A_{c,b}(\theta, t) = A_b(\theta, 0)[\lambda_c/\lambda_b - \lambda_c)](e^{-\lambda_c^t} - e^{-\lambda_b^t}) \quad (2.4)$$

$$A_{c,c}(\theta, t) = A_c(\theta, 0)e^{-\lambda}ct. \quad (2.5)$$

At the second step of derivation, we will use the same Eqs. (2.1) and (2.2) in order to find correlation between the activity on the filter after sampling and concentration in the air.

Expressions for the activity of RaA, RaB, and RaC at the time of the end of filtration ($t = 0$) $A_a(\theta, 0)$, $A_b(\theta, 0)$, $A_c(\theta, 0)$ were obtained by applying the solution for the chain of radioactive transformation when the maternal isotope is long-lived. Each of the decay products is deposited at the constant rate $q_i vk/\lambda_i$, which corresponds to the decay rate of the long-lived maternal nuclide.

$$A_a(\theta, 0) = aq_a vk/\lambda_a(1 - e^{-\lambda_a^\theta}) \quad (2.6)$$

$$A_b(\theta, 0) = avk\{q_a/\lambda_a(1 + (\lambda_b e^{-\lambda_a^\theta} - \lambda_a e^{-\lambda_b^\theta})/(\lambda_a - \lambda_b) + q_b/\lambda_b(1 - e^{-\lambda_b^\theta})\} \quad (2.7)$$

$$A_c(\theta, 0) = avk[q_a\xi_a(\theta) + q_b\xi_b(\theta) + q_c\xi_c(\theta)], \quad (2.8)$$

where

$$\xi_a(\theta) = 1/\lambda_a[1 - \lambda_b\lambda_c \cdot e^{-\lambda_a^\theta}/(\lambda_b - \lambda_a)(\lambda_c - \lambda_a)$$
$$- \lambda_a\lambda_c \cdot e^{-\lambda_b^\theta}/(\lambda_a - \lambda_b)(\lambda_c - \lambda_b) - \lambda_a\lambda_b \cdot e^{-\lambda_c^\theta}/(\lambda_a - \lambda_c(\lambda_b -)_c)] \quad (2.9)$$

$$\xi_b(\theta) = 1/\lambda_b[1 + (\lambda_c e^{-\lambda_b^\theta} - \lambda_b e^{-\lambda_c^\theta})/(\lambda_b - \lambda_c)] \quad (2.10)$$

$$\xi_c(\theta) = 1/\lambda_c \times (1 - e^{-\lambda_c^\theta}) \quad (2.11)$$

$a = 2.22 \times 10^{12}$ decay/min for 1 Ci.

Finally,

$$A_c(\theta, t) = A_{c,a}(\theta, t) + A_{c,b}(\theta, t) + A_{c,c}(\theta, t)$$
$$= avk[q_a\Phi_{a,c}(\theta, t) + q_b\Phi_{b,c}(\theta, t) + q_c\Phi_{c,c}(\theta, t)] \quad (2.12)$$

Similarly, the expression for $A_b(\theta, t)$,

$$A_b(\theta, t) = avk[q_a\Phi_{a,b}(\theta, t) + q_b\Phi_{b,b}(\theta, t)] \quad (2.13)$$

And for $A_a(\theta, t)$,

$$A_a(\theta, t) = avkq_a\Phi_a(\theta, t) \quad (2.14)$$

The final expression for the alpha activity of ^{218}Po (RaA) and ^{218}Po (RaC′) on the filter (i.e., lungs) is

$$A_\alpha = avk\{q_a[\Phi_a(\theta, t) + \Phi_{a,c}(\theta, t)] + q_b\Phi_{b,c}(\theta, t) + q_c\Phi_{c,c}(\theta, t)\}. \quad (2.15)$$

And respectively for the beta-, and gamma-activity of RaB and RaC,

$$A_{\beta,\gamma} = avk\{q_a[\Phi_{a,b}(\theta, t) + \Phi_{a,c}(\theta, t)] + q_b[\Phi_{b,b}(\theta, t) + \Phi_{b,c}(\theta, t)]$$
$$+ q_c\Phi_{c,c}(\theta, t)\}. \quad (2.16)$$

2.3 The General Activity Methods of Measuring Concentration of Radon Decay Products

The first method for the concentration of radon decay products measurement was published in by Tsivoglou (1953). The premise of this method was in analysis of the curve of radioactive decay after sampling is concluded. To determine the three unknown quantities

q_a, q_b, and q_c, the values of the total radioactivity are measured at three different times: 5, 15, and 30 min.

In Kuznets (1956) and Holeidy (1961), another approach was presented, which does not require individual determination of the atmospheric concentration of ^{218}Po (RaA), ^{214}Pb (RaB), and ^{214}Bi (RaC). As a characteristic of the contamination of the atmosphere with the radon decay products, the concept of the potential alpha energy concentration (PAEC) was proposed, which is the energy produced in complete alpha decay, resulting in production of ^{210}Pb (RaD), of all the short-lived radon decay products contained in the unite volume of the air. The maximum permissible value of PAEC may be taken to be 3.8×10^4 Mev/l, corresponding to the equilibrium percentage of the radon decay products at concentration of 1100 Bq/m^3.

A completely self-contained portable sample counter, the TM372 has been the workhorse for radon progeny measurements in Canadian uranium mines for over 20 years. A pump (not included) is used to draw air through a filter, trapping radon progeny on the filter. The filter is then inserted into the TM372 and the alpha radioactivity is counted. A technician uses a known formula to convert the number of counts to working levels (WL).

A technician will typically walk through the work place, taking one sample with his pump and counting the previous sample in the TM372, which he/she carries on a shoulder strap. Using this method, a skilled technician can take a sample every 6 min, which is about three times faster than automated instruments.

Another advantage of TM372 over more complicated instruments is the traceability of the measurements and quality control. Radon progeny measurements are often taken to demonstrate regulatory compliance. It is therefore important that the reported values are traceable. The efficiency of the TM372 can be determined using a traceable source. The flow rate of the sampling pump can be measured on a primary standard, such as a bubble tube. The sampling time is measured with a stopwatch, which can be checked against other watches. The airborne radioactivity readings are then calculated using first principles and traceable input parameters.

More recently, the TM372 has also become the instrument of choice for counting Long Lived Radioactive Dust (LLRD) samples.

To satisfy the conditions in mines where the rapid assessment of results is sometimes more important than the accuracy of the measurement, Markov et al. (1965) and Markov et al. (1962) presented a different variant of the method of the measurement of the general alpha activity, called the "express method." The express method allows the very quick determination (within 10 min) of the concentration of each radon decay product and potential alpha energy concentration with an accuracy of 20–40%, which is completely acceptable for dosimetric purposes. In this method, the 5 min circulation time and the measurement of the alpha activity twice, once from the 1st to the 4th minute, and again from the 7th to the 10th minute after conclusion of the sampling was proposed. The formulas for determining each q and PAEC are

$$q_{\mathrm{a}} = 1.18(n_1 - n_2)/ekv!0^{-10}\ \mathrm{Ci/m^3} \tag{2.17}$$

$$q_{\mathrm{b}} = 3n_2/ekv10^{-11}\ \mathrm{Ci/m^3} \tag{2.18}$$

$$q_{\mathrm{c}} = (5.97n_1 - 2.44n_2)/ekv10^{-11}\ \mathrm{Ci/m^3} \tag{2.19}$$

$$\mathrm{PAEC} = 40n_2/ekv\ \mathrm{Mev/l.} \tag{2.20}$$

The authors also pointed out that the 5 min sampling time is not mandatory for this method. In the case when the slightly lower accuracy of the PAEC measurements is acceptable the time of the PAEC determination can be decreased using formula

$$\mathrm{PAEC} = mn/ekv.$$

2.4 Measurement of Radon Decay Products in Air by Alpha and Beta Spectrometry

The methods described above were used, for example, for daily monitoring in the atmosphere of underground mining operations. In such situations, the monitoring equipment must be portable, light, simple to operate, and capable of functioning in considerable gamma fields. High accuracy is often not required for this equipment.

All methods of determining the concentrations of each radon decay product, based on measurement of total alpha radioactivity collected on a filter, can have substantial errors (Nazaroff, 1988; Ruzer, 1997).

Although the health effects associated with radon decay products' exposures do not critically depend upon the ratio of the ^{218}Po and ^{214}Po concentrations, in some cases, high inherent accuracy in the measurement of radon decay products is important, such as in

1. the study of the behavior of aerosols, including the attached and unattached fraction of radon decay products,
2. examination of the correlation between the ventilation rate and the shift of equilibrium,
3. standardization and calibration of decay product measurements.

Practically, in many cases determining the dose due to the unattached radon decay products will require that airborne concentration of ^{214}Pb and ^{214}Bi be accurately measured. Even though their concentrations may be lower than that of ^{218}Po, their indirect effect on the dose, as estimated by the potential alpha energy concentration (PAEC), can be substantial due to ^{218}Po alone. Thus, the accuracy afforded by alpha spectrometry may make it the preferred measurement method.

In some practical situations such as high aerosol (dust) concentration or high humidity, the results of the measurements can be distorted due to the absorption of alpha radiation by the aerosols or the water on the filter. The method, which will be present below, of determining of ^{218}Po, ^{214}Pb, and ^{214}Bi (^{214}Po) in air based on the measurement of the activity on the filter using both alpha and beta spectrometry permits assessment of the effect of absorption of the alpha radiation with high accuracy (Ruzer et al., 1964).

2.4.1 *Measurement Procedure and Experimental Results*

The short-lived alpha emitters in the ^{222}Rn series are ^{218}Po and ^{214}Po with alpha particles energy of 6.00 and 7.6 MeV, respectively; the short-lived beta emitters are ^{214}Pb and ^{214}Bi with the maximum (endpoint) beta energies of 1.024 and 3.27 MeV, respectively. In the former case, the strongest beta decay transitions have endpoint energies of 0.67 (48%) and 0.73 (42%). As a result

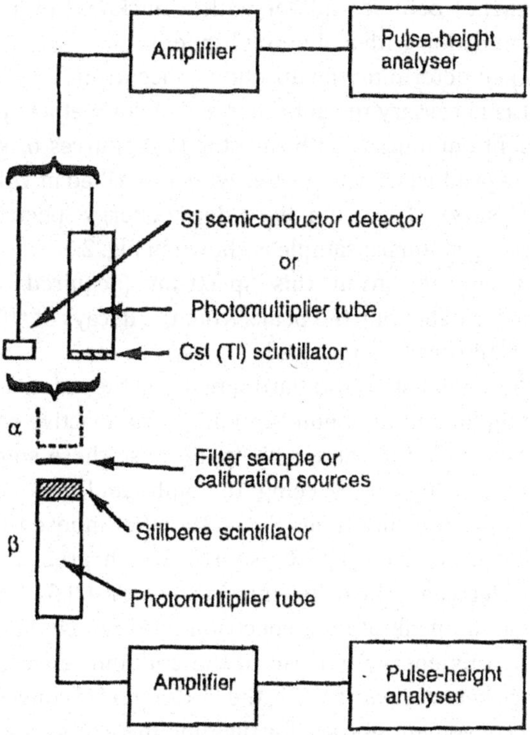

Figure 2.1 Block diagram of detectors used for the measurement of alpha and beta particles. Republished with permission of Taylor and Francis Group LLC Books, from *Aerosols Handbook: Measurement, Dosimetry, and Health Effects*, Lev S. Ruzer, 201; permission conveyed through Copyright Clearance Center, Inc.

of the considerable difference between the energies for either alpha or beta emissions from these nuclides, high-energy resolution detection methods are not needed and the activity of the progeny on the filter can be relatively easily measured separately by means of scintillation detectors. The equipment used for these measurements is shown in Fig. 2.1.

Alpha particle counting was done with either a 0.1 mm-thick Cs(Tl) scintillator coupled to a multiplier tube or a Si semiconductor detector, with alpha particle energy resolutions of 9% and 1%, respectively. For measuring the beta spectra, a stilbene (1,2-

diphenylethene) beta scintillator with a thickness of 13 mm was used in conjunction with a photomultiplier tube.

In order to determine the absolute concentration of each decay product, it is necessary to calibrate the detection efficiencies of the measurement equipment with the standard sources of short-lived radon decay products. Such sources were described in Volkova et al. (1966) and Ruzer (1993). An alpha decay energy spectrum from a non-emanating standard sample is shown in Fig. 2.2.

As can be seen from this spectrum (acquired with a Si semiconductor detector), the peaks from the decays of ^{226}Ra, ^{222}Rn, ^{218}Po, and ^{214}Po are well resolved.

In this non-emanating standard sample, all the radon decay products (both alpha and beta emitters) are in radioactive equilibrium and therefore have the same activity. Because these sources were mounted on the thin foil backing, the alpha and beta spectra can be acquired at the same time (Fig. 2.3); superimposed on Fig. 2.3 are data collected from a ^{137}Cs source, which produces internal conversion electrons. The main emission peak is at 0.624 MeV, which accounts for the peak of beta spectrum between channels 20 and 25. Because this energy is close to the endpoint energies for the most intense beta decays of ^{214}Pb, the ^{137}Cs internal conversion peak provides a convenient marker for dividing the energy spectrum for the beta decays from the ^{222}Rn decay products ^{214}Pb and ^{214}Bi.

Using the non-emanating standard sample to provide detection efficiencies and measuring the air flow rate through the sampling filter, all activity measurements can be converted directly into airborne activity concentrations (Bq per volume of the air). For these experiments, airborne radon decay products were collected by pumping a specified volume of air at a rate of 20 l/min from the test chamber through a fiber filter especially designed for alpha spectrometry (filter type LFS). Measurement of the alpha activity from the front (collection) side of the filter and beta activity from the back of the filter were done simultaneously.

In order to determine the ^{214}Pb and ^{214}Bi concentrations, the ^{137}Cs source of monoenergetic inner conversion electrons, noted earlier, was used to find the edge of the ^{214}Pb beta spectrum. Since all but 10% of the ^{214}Pb decays have maximum beta decay energies <0.73 MeV, it is assumed that all electrons with energies higher

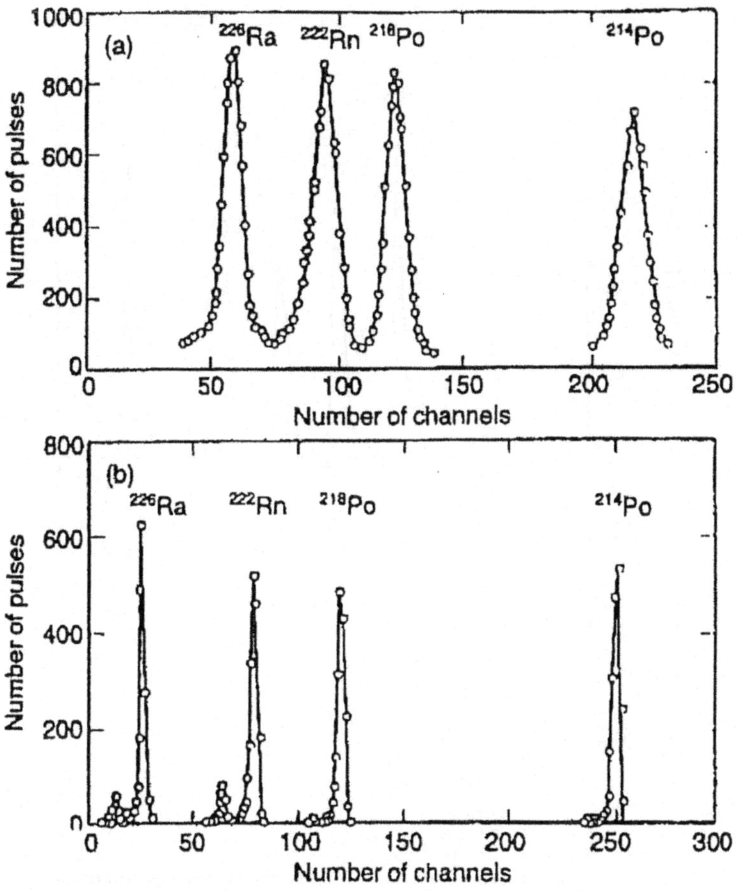

Figure 2.2 Alpha spectra from a ^{222}Rn series non-emanating sample. Copyright (2012). From *Aerosols Handbook: Measurement, Dosimetry, and Health Effects, Second Edition,* edited by Lev S. Ruzer and Naomi H. Harley. Reproduced by permission of Taylor and Francis Group, LLC, a division of Informa plc.

than this 0.73 MeV edge are due to the beta decay of ^{214}Bi, while that portion of the energy spectrum with energies below this value consists of beta decays from both ^{214}Pb and ^{214}Bi. Based on the usual beta decays from energy distribution, it is reasonable to neglect the small number of beta particles from ^{214}Pb with energies greater than 0.73 MeV. A comparison of the integrated beta decays with energies

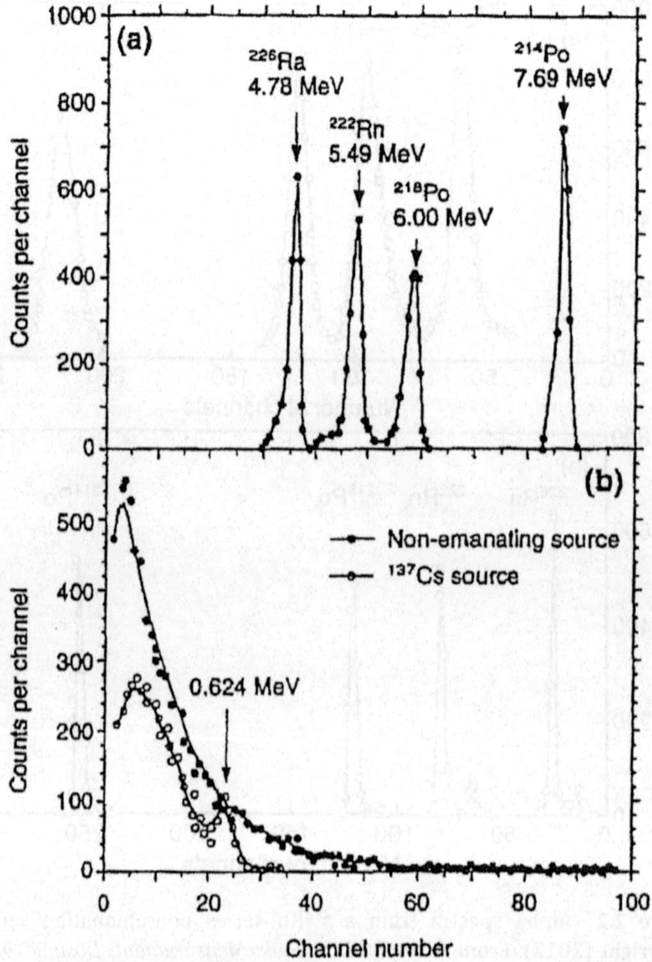

Figure 2.3 Alpha and beta spectra from non-emanating standard source (a). Alpha spectra from non-emanating acquired with a semiconductor detector. Copyright (2012). From *Aerosols Handbook: Measurement, Dosimetry, and Health Effects, Second Edition*, edited by Lev S. Ruzer and Naomi H. Harley. Reproduced by permission of Taylor and Francis Group, LLC, a division of Informa plc.

above 0.73 MeV obtained from the non-emanating standard source with that from the filter sample permits the direct determination of the ^{214}Bi activity. A similar procedure for the total beta decays with energies lower than 0.73 MeV provides the combined ^{214}Pb and ^{214}Bi activities on the filter sample. The ^{214}Pb activity can be obtained by simple subs traction of the ^{214}Bi activity from the combined activity.

2.5 Absorption of Alpha Radiation in the sample

Using the technique described above to provide an independent measurement of both ^{214}Bi and ^{214}Po on the filter (Labushkin et al., 1965), one can then evaluate the apparent loss of alpha activity due to self-absorption in thick filter samples. The coefficient of absorption is defined as the fractional difference between the actual ^{214}Po alpha activity on the filter and the measured ^{214}Po activity, corrected for detector efficiencies:

$$k(m) = 1 - A_2/A_1, \tag{2.21}$$

where $k(m)$ is the absorption coefficient as a function of collected aerosol mass (mg·cm^{-2}), A_2 is the measured ^{214}Po alpha activity on the filter, and $A_1$is the actual ^{214}Po alpha activity collected on the filter. Due to the very short half-life of ^{214}Po, the alpha activity of this nuclide is identical to the beta activity of its precursor, ^{214}Bi. Thus, assuming adsorption of beta particles can be neglected, measurement of the betas from ^{214}Bi can be used to determine A_1:

$$A_1 = N_1(\beta)/e_\beta \tag{2.22}$$

and

$$A_2 = N_2(\alpha)/e_\alpha, \tag{2.23}$$

where $N_1(\beta)$ is the beta count rate for ^{214}Bi and $N_2(\alpha)$ is the alpha count rate for ^{214}Po. The quantities e_β and e_α are the detection efficiencies for the alpha and beta radiation, respectively. These can be determined directly from measurements using the non-emanating standard source:

$$A_0 = N_0(\alpha)/e_\alpha = N_0(\beta)/e_\beta, \tag{2.24}$$

where A_0 is the activity of ^{214}Po in non-emanating standard source (which is also the ^{214}Bi activity of that source) and $N_0(\alpha)$ and $N_0(\beta)$ are the count rates for the alpha decays from ^{214}Po and the beta decay from ^{214}Bi, respectively. In principle, the detection efficiencies for both alpha and beta particles are energy dependent. Any energy dependence can be evaluated by using the non-emanating source.

Substituting in Eq. 2.21, we have formula for the absorption coefficient in terms of measured quantities:

$$\begin{aligned} k(m) &= 1 - N_2(\alpha)/e_\alpha/N_1(\beta)/e_\beta \\ &= 1 - N_2 e_\beta/N_1 e_\alpha \cdot [k(m) = 1 - A_2/A_1] \end{aligned} \quad (2.25)$$

In this work, the non-emanating standard source had a ^{226}Ra activity of 44 Bq and had the same geometry as the filter.

Experiments were performed to study the correlation between the mass of aerosol collected and the self-absorption of the alpha radiation of the activity deposited on the filter. The distortion of the alpha particle spectrum was studied and, using the measured sampling air flow rates, a method for assessment of the aerosol concentration in the air was proposed based on the measurement activity of ^{214}Bi and ^{214}Po (Ruzer et al., 1964). The coefficient of absorption of the alpha activity of ^{214}Po in the filter samples was measured for aerosol mass collected on the filter ranging in thickness from 0 to 18 mg·cm^{-2}.

For these experiments, NH_4Cl aerosols were generated by gas-phase condensation from the gas-phase interaction $HCL + NH_3 = NH_4Cl$. The aerosols were generated in a 2 m^3 chamber.

Radon was then injected into the chamber. Following the establishment of radioactive equilibrium between radon and its decay products, filter samples were collected using the fiber filter developed for alpha spectrometry noted previously increased. These alpha particles counted and thus increasing the proportion of the high-energy alpha particles counted.

As has been shown, the problem of collecting a sample of airborne activity can compound the analytical difficulties due to the need to sample large quantities of air, which may contain significant concentrations of inactive (non-radioactive) aerosol. This material, when collected on the filter along with the radon decay products, may distort the alpha spectra due to adsorption.

The method described here can be used to correct the measurements.

The use of a non-emanating reference standard as part of this process has several advantages. First, it provides a source of both alpha and beta particles with exact same energies as are observed in the measurement of radon decay product samples, so that detector efficiencies as a function of energy can be precisely obtained. Second, the source provides both the alpha and beta particles with essentially the same geometry as the filter samples, so no further correction needed. Third, the non-emanating source provided a tool for checking the linearity of the spectrometer across the wide range of energies needed for alpha spectrometric measurements of Rn decay products. Even higher alpha energies can be obtained by using a non-emanating sample of ^{228}Th, where one of the ^{212}Bi alpha peaks has the energy of 8.78 MeV.

2.6 Measurement Procedure for Determination of Activity of RaA, RaB, RaC, and RaC′ on Filter by Alpha and Beta Spectrometry (Labushkin, 1965; Ruzer et al., 1964)

2.6.1 *^{218}Po (RaA) Activity Measurement*

As we can see in Fig. 2.4, the division of RaA and RaC′ presents no difficulties even if we use the scintillation spectrometer. Let us denote by A_0 the activity of ^{226}Ra in the standard non-emanating source. Due to equilibrium in this source activity of ^{222}Rn, ^{218}Po and ^{214}Po will also be A_0. When taking the measurements, the width of the window of the differential discriminator should be such that it can count only the pulses from RaA. The width and exact location of the window should be chosen by means of the non-emanating sample.

Let us denote the following:

1. $N_{a,o}$: count rate of RaA corresponded to the width and location of the window of the alpha-spectrometer in measuring the non-emanating source

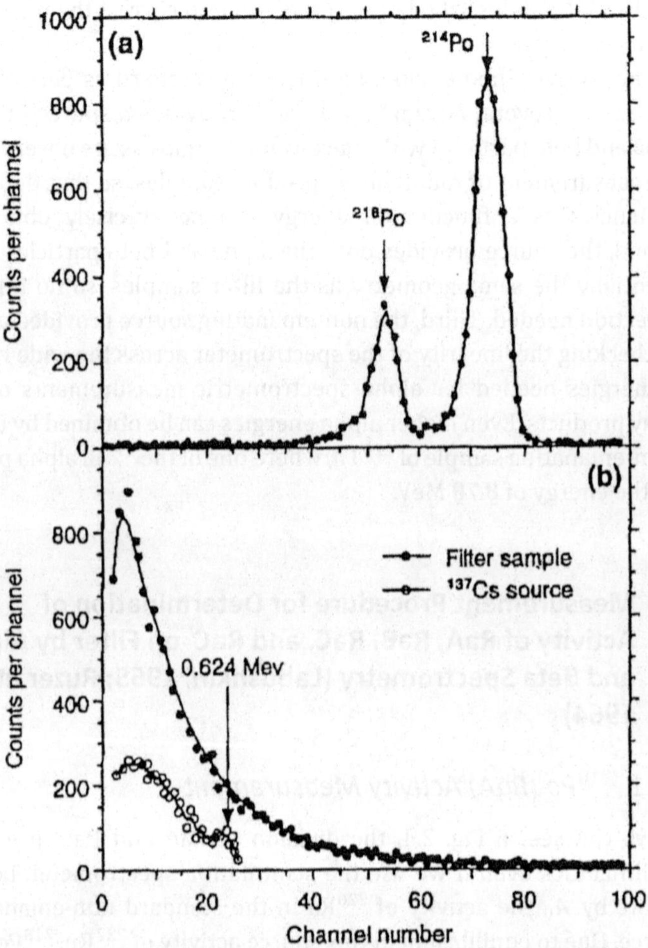

Figure 2.4 Spectra acquired from a filter sample of radon progeny. Copyright (2012). From *Aerosols Handbook: Measurement, Dosimetry, and Health Effects*, Second Edition, edited by Lev S. Ruzer and Naomi H. Harley. Reproduced by permission of Taylor and Francis Group, LLC, a division of Informa plc.

2. N_a: count rate of RaA corresponded to the width and location in measuring of the filter
3. n_a: number of pulses for the time of measurement of the filter of the activity of RaA at the time t after sampling conclusion.

Then

$$N_0 = e_\alpha A_0 \text{ and } N_a = e_\alpha A_a(\theta, t) \tag{2.26}$$

and number of the pulses from RaA on the filter n_a

$$n_a e^{-\lambda_a^t} dt = N_a(1 - e^{-\lambda_a^t})/\lambda_a \tag{2.27}$$

and consequently from the previous two equations

$$A_a(\theta, t) = A_{0N_a}/N_0 = A_{0n_a}\lambda_a/N_{a,0}(1 - e^{-\lambda_a^t}). \tag{2.28}$$

In this case it is not important at what exactly moment the determination of the A_a takes place because by the means of the exponential factor, we can calculate activity for the every time and for the completion of sampling as well:

$$A_a(\theta, 0) = A_a(\theta, t)e^{\lambda}a^t. \tag{2.29}$$

Of course, in these measurements as in other measurements, all geometric differences should be minimal.

2.6.2 ^{214}Po (RaC′) Activity Measurement

The activity of the RaC′ on the filter is measured in a similar manner. In this case, it is not necessary to use the differential discriminator, the integral discriminator can be used in the way to discriminate all pulses with the energy a little higher than energy of alpha particles of the RaA. Due to the fact that contribution in the count rate of RaC′ on the filter is not only by RaC but also by RaA and RaB, the correlation between the activity of the RaC on the filter for different time cannot be established in the same simple way as that for RaA. Therefore in the case of RaC′, it is better to decrease as much as possible the duration of the measurement. As it is clear from Figs. 2.5 and 2.6, in the cases when the shift of equilibrium is not so big the activity of the RaC on the filter in the first minutes after sampling completion do not change substantially, which permit to increase the duration of the measurement to achieve the lower statistical error. In the case of the substantial shift of equilibrium, the curves in Figs. 2.5 and 2.6 allow us to assess the maximum error and to choose the necessary duration of the measurement for achieving the appropriate accuracy of measurement. The activity of the RaC′ on the filter can be determined according to the following formula:

$$A_{c'}(\theta, t) = A_0 N_{c'}/N_0 \tag{2.30}$$

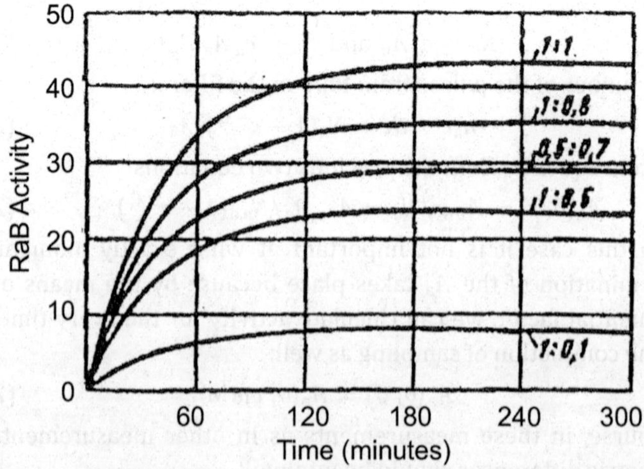

Figure 2.5 Dependency of RaB activity on duration of filtration for various values of q_A:q_B. Copyright (2012). From *Aerosols Handbook: Measurement, Dosimetry, and Health Effects*, Second Edition, edited by Lev S. Ruzer and Naomi H. Harley. Reproduced by permission of Taylor and Francis Group, LLC, a division of Informa plc.

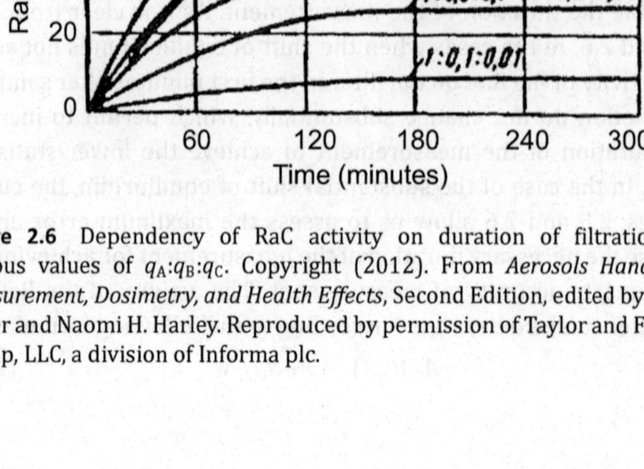

Figure 2.6 Dependency of RaC activity on duration of filtration for various values of q_A:q_B:q_C. Copyright (2012). From *Aerosols Handbook: Measurement, Dosimetry, and Health Effects*, Second Edition, edited by Lev S. Ruzer and Naomi H. Harley. Reproduced by permission of Taylor and Francis Group, LLC, a division of Informa plc.

2.6.3 ^{214}Pb (RaC) Activity Measurement

The division of the RaB and RaC in the beta spectra is not so obvious as for alpha spectra of RaA and RaC′ due to the fact that beta spectra is indiscrete. It was possible to overcome these difficulties for two reasons. First, the maximum energies of beta spectra of RaB and RaC differ substantially from one another. Second, the monoenergetic line of the electrons of the inner conversion of the ^{137}Cs corresponds to the edge between RaB and RaC. Therefore for the RaC activity on the filter determination, it is necessary first to establish the integral discriminator threshold in such a way that detector will count only pulses with the energy larger than that for source of the monoenergetic electrons of ^{137}Cs conversion with the very thin foil. If $N_{c,o}$ is the count rate of RaC from the non-emanating source with the background with chosen discriminator threshold, N_c is the count rate of RaC on the filter with the same background and discriminator threshold and N_{bg} the count rate for the same discriminator threshold; then the activity of RaC on the filter is

$$A_c(\theta, t) = A_0(N_c - N_{bg})/(N_{c,o} - N_{bg}). \tag{2.31}$$

What was mentioned about the correlation of the activity of the RaC′ on the filter in different moments of time is true for RaC.

2.6.4 ^{214}Bi (RaB) Activity Measurement

The RaB activity on the filter is measured by subtraction of the count rate of RaC from the summary count rate of RaB + RaC. Let us denote the following:

1. $N_{b+c,0}$: the count rate from the standard non-emanating source with the background
2. N_{b+c}: count rate from RaB + RaC on the filter with the background
3. N_{bg}: background count rate

Then the counts rates of RaB in the standard source $N_{b,o}$ and on the filter N_b will be

$$\begin{aligned} N_{b,o} &= (N_{b+c,0} - N_{bg}) - (N_{c,0} - N_{bg}) \\ &= (N_{b+c} - N_{bg}) - (N_c - N_{bg}) \end{aligned} \tag{2.32}$$

and the activity of the RaB on the filter will be

$$A_b(\theta, t) = A_0 N_b/N_{b,o} = A_0[(N_{b+c} - N_{bg}) \\ -(N_c - N_{bg})]/[(N_{b+c,0} - N_{bg}) - (N_{c,0} - N_{bg})]. \quad (2.33)$$

Since the expression for $A_b(\theta, t)$ consists of two factors, one of which is determined by the activity of the RaA, it is possible to establish correlation between the activities of RaB in different moments of time.

Transfer from the measured activities of each decay product on the filter to the corresponding concentration should be made according the following formulas:

$$q_a = [N_a(\theta, t)/N_{a,o}]A_0/vk\Phi_a(\theta, t) \quad (2.34)$$

$$q_b = A_0/vk\Phi_{b,b}(\theta, t)\{[N_b(\theta, t)/N_{b,o}] \\ - [N_a(\theta, t)/N_{a,o}] - [\Phi_{a,b}(\theta, t)/\Phi_a(\theta, t)]\} \quad (2.35)$$

$$q_c = A_0/vk\Phi_{c,c}(\theta, t)\{\{[N_c(\theta, t)/N_{c,o}] \\ - [N_b(\theta, t)/N_{b,o}][\Phi_{b,c}(\theta, t)/\Phi_{b,b}(\theta, t)]\} \\ - [N_a(\theta, t)/N_{a,o}]\{[\Phi_{a,c}(\theta, t)/\Phi_a(\theta, t)] \\ + [\Phi_{b,c}(\theta, t)/\Phi_{b,b}(\theta, t)] \times [\Phi_{a,b}(\theta, t)/\Phi_a(\theta, t)]\}\} \quad (2.36)$$

The values for the functions $\Phi_{i,j}(\theta, t)$ for different θ and t are presented in Table 2.1 (Ruzer et al., 2004). For example, for $\theta = 5$ min and $t = 1$ min and the duration of the measurement 1 min,

$$q_a = 0.032 A_0 N_a/N_{a,o} \quad (2.37)$$

$$q_b = A_0[(0.0115 N_b/N_{b,o}) - 0.0028 N_a/N_{a,o}] \quad (2.38)$$

$$q_c = A_0[(0.0115 N_c/N_{c,o}) - 0.0023 N_b/N_{b,o} - 0.0009 N_a/N_{a,o}]. \quad (2.39)$$

2.7 Characteristics of Thoron and Actinon Decay Products

As can be seen in Fig. 2.7, the difference between the chain of thoron from radon shows that the half-lives of Tn and ^{216}Po (ThA) are small. In fact, the whole thorium series contains no long-lived isotopes. For dosimetry purposes, the four isotopes ^{212}Pb (ThB), ^{212}Bi (ThC), ^{212}Po (ThC′) and ^{208}Tl (ThC″) are of primary interest. ThA is not usually taken into consideration because of its short half-life.

Table 2.1 Values of $\Phi_{b,b}(\theta, t)\Phi_{b,c}(\theta, t)$ and $\Phi_{c,c}(\theta, t)$ for thoron progeny

θ	$\Phi_{i,j}$	$\Phi_{i,j}$ for t (min)						
		0	5	10	15	30	60	180
	$\Phi_{b,b}$	5.0	5.0	4.93	4.91	4.83	4.67	4.10
5	$\Phi_{b,c}$	0.14	0.41	0.66	0.90	1.53	2.46	3.85
	$\Phi_{c,c}$	4.86	4.59	4.33	4.09	3.45	2.44	0.62
	$\Phi_{b,b}$	9.95	9.90	9.84	9.79	9.63	9.32	8.18
10	$\Phi_{b,c}$	0.55	1.07	1.56	2.02	3.23	5.05	7.71
	$\Phi_{c,c}$	9.45	8.92	8.38	7.92	6.67	4.73	1.20
	$\Phi_{b,b}$	14.9	14.8	14.7	14.64	14.4	13.9	12.2
	$\Phi_{b,c}$	1.20	1.96	2.68	3.34	5.11	7.74	11.55
15	$\Phi_{c,c}$	13.8	13.0	12.3	11.6	9.77	6.93	1.76
	$\Phi_{b,b}$	29.5	29.4	29.2	29.0	28.6	27.65	24.3
	$\Phi_{b,c}$	4.56	5.95	6.55	8.46	11.7	16.4	23.2
	$\Phi_{c,c}$	25.4	24.0	22.6	21.4	18.0	12.8	3.23
	$\Phi_{b,b}$	58.1	57.8	57.5	57.1	56.2	54.4	47.7
60	$\Phi_{b,c}$	16.2	18.6	20.7	22.8	28.1	36.0	46.7
	$\Phi_{c,c}$	43.4	41.0	38.7	36.55	30.8	21.8	5.52
	$\Phi_{b,b}$	163.4	162.6	161.7	160.8	158.2	153.1	134.3
180	$\Phi_{b,c}$	96.4	100.1	103.6	106.8	115.1	126.8	137.7
	$\Phi_{c,c}$	76.2	72.0	67.9	64.2	54.0	38.3	9.69

Source: Copyright (2012). From *Aerosols Handbook: Measurement, Dosimetry, and Health Effects*, Second Edition, edited by Lev S. Ruzer and Naomi H. Harley. Reproduced by permission of Taylor and Francis Group, LLC, a division of Informa plc.

2.8 The Basic Equations for Thoron and Actinon Series

2.8.1 *Thoron Series*

Let us denote for thoron progeny as in the case of radon decay products: λ_a, λ_b, λ_c, $\lambda_{c'}$, and $\lambda_{c'}$ are decay constants for ThA, ThB, ThC, ThC′, and ThC′, respectively; $A_a(\theta, t)$, $A_b(\theta, t)$, $A_c(\theta, t)$, $A_{c'}(\theta, t)$ and $A_{c'}(\theta, t)$ are the activities in the samples.

Applying the same relationships as for radon, we obtain the expression for the activity on the filter (in the lungs):

$$A_a(\theta, t) = avkq_a\Phi_a(\theta, t) \tag{2.40}$$

$$A_b(\theta, t) = vk[q_a\Phi_{a,b}(\theta, t) + q_b\Phi_{b,b}(\theta, t)] \tag{2.41}$$

$$A_c(\theta, t) = vk[q_a\Phi_{a,c}(\theta, t) + q_b\Phi_{b,c}(\theta, t) + q_c\Phi_{c,c}(\theta, t)] \tag{2.42}$$

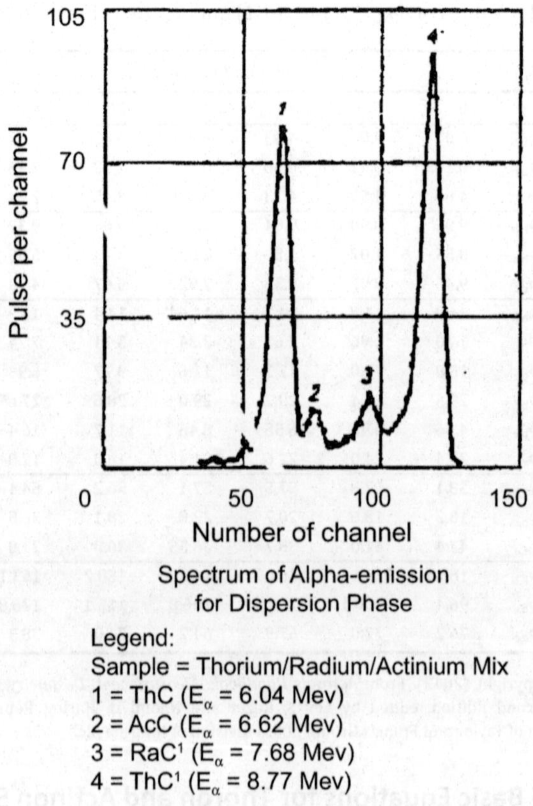

Figure 2.7 Spectra from sample thorium/radium/actinium mix. Copyright (2012). From *Aerosols Handbook: Measurement, Dosimetry, and Health Effects*, Second Edition, edited by Lev S. Ruzer and Naomi H. Harley. Reproduced by permission of Taylor and Francis Group, LLC, a division of Informa plc.

$$A'_c(\theta, t) = 0.663A_c(\theta, t) \tag{2.43}$$

Because the contribution of ThA in the activity of ThB and ThC is very small ($\Phi_{a,b}(\theta, t) = 0$ and $\Phi_{b,b}(\theta, t) = 0$), the equations can be rewritten as follows:

$$A_b(\theta, t) = vkq_b\Phi_{b,b}(\theta, t)] \tag{2.44}$$

$$A_c(\theta, t) = vk[q_b\Phi_{b,c}(\theta, t) + q_c\Phi_{c,c}(\theta, t)] \tag{2.45}$$

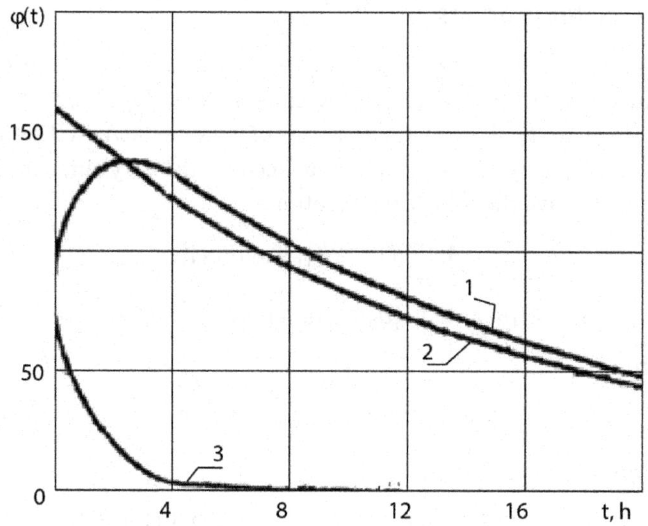

Figure 2.8 Graphs of the functions of $\Phi_{i,j}(\theta, t)$. Copyright (2012). From *Aerosols Handbook: Measurement, Dosimetry, and Health Effects*, Second Edition, edited by Lev S. Ruzer and Naomi H. Harley. Reproduced by permission of Taylor and Francis Group, LLC, a division of Informa plc.

The activities of ThC′ (ThC) measured for the two different moments of time t_1 and t_2 after sampling q_b and q_c can be calculated from the following equations:

$$q_b = 1/kv\{[A_c(\theta, t_1)\Phi_{c,c}(\theta, t_2) - A_c(\theta, t_2)\Phi_{c,c}(\theta, t_1)]/ [\Phi_{b,c}(\theta, t_1)\Phi_{c,c}(\theta, t_2) - \Phi_{b,c}(\theta, t_2)\Phi_{c,c}(\theta, t_1)]\} \quad (2.46)$$

$$q_c = 1/kv\{[A_c(\theta, t_2)\Phi_{b,c}(\theta, t_2) - A_c(\theta, t_1)\Phi_{b,c}(\theta, t_1)]/ [\Phi_{b,c}(\theta, t_2)\Phi_{c,c}(\theta, t_1) - \Phi_{b,c}(\theta, t_1)\Phi_{c,c}(\theta, t_2)]\} \quad (2.47)$$

Graphs of the functions of $\Phi_{i,j}(\theta, t)$ are presented in Fig. 2.8 (see Ruzer et al., 2004).

The values of the functions $\Phi_{i,j}(\theta, t)$ for different θ and t are presented in Table 2.1, which allows to calculate the concentrations of ThB and ThC.

2.8.2 *Actinon Series*

Let us denote for actinon progeny as in the case of radon decay products: λ_a, λ_b, and λ_c are decay constants, and q_a, q_b, q_c, q_c, and $A_a(\theta, t)$, $A_b(\theta, t)$, $A_c(\theta, t)$ are activities of isotopes AcA, AcB, and AcC on the filter, respectively. Taking into account the very small half-live of RaA, we have the following equations:

$$A_b(\theta, t) = vkq_b\Phi_{b,b}(\theta, t)] \tag{2.48}$$

$$A_c(\theta, t) = vk[q_b\Phi_{b,c}(\theta, t) + q_c\Phi_{c,c}(\theta, t)], \tag{2.49}$$

where

$$\Phi_{b,b}(\theta, t)] = 1/\lambda_b(1 - e^{-\lambda_b^\theta})e^{-\lambda_b^\theta} \tag{2.50}$$

$$\Phi_{b,c}(\theta, t) = 1/\lambda_b\{[1 + (\lambda_c e^{-\lambda_b^\theta} - \lambda_b e^{-\lambda_c^\theta})/(\lambda_b - \lambda_c)]e^{-\lambda_c^t} + 1/\lambda_b(1 - e^{-\lambda_b^\theta})\lambda_c(e^{-\lambda_c^\theta} - e^{-\lambda_b^\theta})/(\lambda_b - \lambda_c)\} \tag{2.51}$$

$$\Phi_{c,c}(\theta, t) = 1/\lambda_c(1 - e^{-\lambda_c^\theta})e^{-\lambda_c\theta} (2.52) \tag{2.52}$$

We can get similar equations for $A_{c'}$. As for the concentration of each decay product, it is better to determine it for the alpha emitter AcC with alpha particles energy of 6.56 MeV.

As in the case of radon decay product series, the most accurate method of the measurements of decay products in air is spectrometry. This method for thoron and actinon decay products series was described in Zhivet'ev (1966).

For the alpha spectrometry of thoron and radon decay products measurements, the similar non-emanating samples consisting of radiothorium (^{228}Th) mixed with actinium (^{227}Ac) and consequently with all of their decay products were developed. All of these non-emanating sources were developed as a cooperative effort between the All-Union Institute of Physico-Technical and Radiotechnical Measurements in Moscow and the Radium Institute in Leningrad (USSR). Each sample consists of a backing, either a foil or a thick metal blank, onto which is deposited the appropriate long-lived parent radionuclide (^{226}Ra, ^{228}Th, ^{227}Ac) in a solution that is then evaporated. This is then sealed by deposition of a 0.2 μm layer, which retains Rn with the efficiency nominally greater than 99.9%, (i.e., that after more than 3 years only 0.1% Rn emanated from the

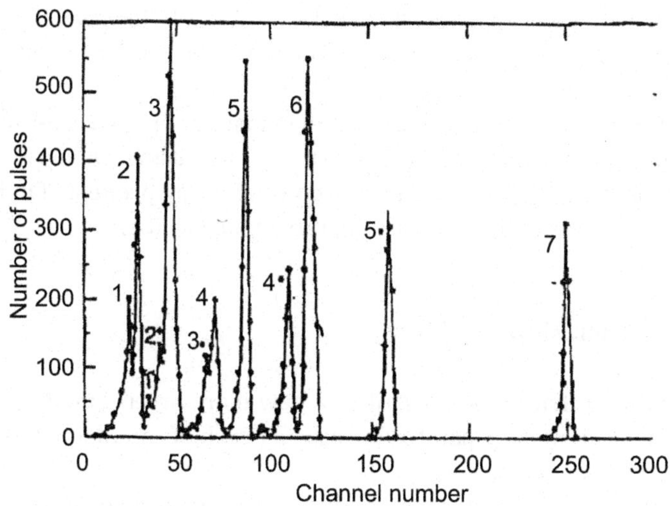

Figure 2.9 Alpha spectrum from a ^{220}Rn and ^{219}Rn series sample obtained using a semiconductor detector. The numbered peaks correspond to the following α particles. In the ^{228}Th (^{220}Rn) series, peaks 1 and 2, 5.34 and 5.42 MeV (from ^{228}Th); peak 3, 5.45 and 5.69 MeV (^{224}Ra); peak 3, 5.45 and 5.69 MeV (^{224}Ra); peak 4, 6.05 MeV (^{212}Bi); peak 5, 6.29 MeV (^{220}Rn); peak 6, 6.78 MeV (^{216}Po), and peak 7, 8.78 MeV (^{212}Po). In the ^{227}Ac (^{219}Rn) series, peaks 1* and 2*, 5.61 and 5.71 MeV (^{223}Ra); peak 3*, 5.90 MeV (^{227}Th); peak 4*, 6.55 MeV (^{211}Bi), and peak 5*, 7.39 MeV (^{215}Po). (Alpha energies here and in text are taken from Browne and Firestone, 1986). Copyright (2012). From *Aerosols Handbook: Measurement, Dosimetry, and Health Effects*, Second Edition, edited by Lev S. Ruzer and Naomi H. Harley. Reproduced by permission of Taylor and Francis Group, LLC, a division of Informa plc.

source). The peak width (FWHM) due to the loss in the source is approximately 50 keV. Samples with activities in the range 40–4000 Bq have been developed with the areas from 5 to 20 cm^2. The alpha spectra for such non-emanating samples for thoron and actinon and its decay products are presented in Fig. 2.9.

The peaks on the alpha spectrum are (1) ThC with the energy of the alpha particles $E_a = 6.04$ MeV; (2) AcC ($E_a = 6.62$ MeV), (3) RaC′ ($E_a = 7.68$ MeV); (4) ThC′ ($E_a = 8.87$ MeV); for thoron decay products, as a result of self-absorption in the dust or the water on the sample, there can be substantial amount of alpha particles with the energy lower than for ThC′ ($E_a = 8.87$ MeV). However, because the closest peak of RaC′ is very far from ThC′, the "tail" from ThC′ can be easily detected.

Another advantage of the non-emanating samples and spectrometric methods is the opportunity for using them in the environment when all three or two of the decay products families are presented in the air, such as in rare metal facilities.

2.9 Conclusion

1. In this chapter, we described a new more precise method and measurement separately measuring each of the radon, thoron, and actinon progeny.
2. We also presented information on the unique radioactive sources for short-lived nuclei with constant activity and inert gas radon (thoron and actinon) in the form of solid (not gaseous) radioactive source.
3. Such sources have broad practical applications in the measurement of radioactivity, including the examination of the linearity of spectrometers.
4. We also presented a new idea and experimental results on the assessment of distortion of alpha spectra due to non-radioactive aerosol or water in the sample.

References

Bateman H (1910) The solution of a system of differential equations occurring in the theory of radioactive transformations, *Proc Cambridge Philos Soc*, **15**, 423–427.

Holeidy (1961).

Kuznets HH (1956) *American Industrial Hygiene Association Quarterly*, **17**(5).

Labushkin VG, Ruzer LS (1965) A method of determining the concentration of the short-lived daughter products of radon in the air by the alpha- and beta-radiations. *Atomic Energy (Atomnaya Energiya)* **19**, 24–28.

Nazaroff WW, Nero AV (eds.) (1988) *Radon and Its Decay Products in Indoor Air*. New York, John Wiley.

Ruzer LS (1958) Calculation of dose of radon inhaled, *Atomnaya Energiya*, 189–194, February.

Ruzer LS (1968) *Radioactive Aerosols*, Moscow (in Russian).

Ruzer LS (1993) Non-emanating samples of the Rn series from 226Ra, 228Th and 227Ac. *Radiation Prot Dosimetry* **46**(2), 127–128.

Ruzer LS, Labushkin VG (1965) The method of determining the concentrations of the short-lived daughter products of radon. Patent No. 171478. *Bull Inventions* **11**, Moscow, USSR (in Russian).

Ruzer LS, Sextro R (1997) Measurement of radon decay products in air by alpha and beta spectrometry. *Radiation Prot Dosimetry* **72**(1), 43–48.

Ruzer L, et al. (1964) The method of determining of the absorbed doses in organism upon inhalation of radon. Patent no. 165250, *Bull Inventions*, **28**, Moscow, USSR (in Russian).

Tsivoglou EC (1953) Quantitative description of successive transformations in atmospheric samples. PhD dissertation, Ohio State University.

Volkova EA, Ziv DU, Labushkin VG, Ruzer LS, Stepanov EK, Tyutikov NV (1966) Defining the parameters of alpha-spectrometers with the help of Ra^{226} and Rd Th isotopes (sources of radiation?). *Equipment Tech Exp* **4**, 36–39.

Zhivet'ev VM, Labushkin VG, Ruzer LS (1966) On measurement of thoron daughter products concentration in air. *Atomnaya Energiya (Atomic Energy)* **20**(6), 511.

Chapter 3

Unattached Activity of Radon Progeny

3.1 Unattached Activity Properties

Several studies published in the 1950s and 1960s noted the particular role of the unattached radioactivity of radon decay products (Knutson, 1988; Hopke, 1989). It was postulated that upon inhalation, the high mobility (large diffusion coefficient) of this radioactivity should cause significant diffusion in the lung airways of such radioactivity and hence the main biological effect of the radiation, to be in trachea. This was, in fact, confirmed when medical researchers observed the localization of lung cancer seen in miners in the respiratory systems of miners. Although the effects of unattached fraction were documented long ago, they are still not fully understood today, especially in connection with the danger of radon in homes. To this day, a few instruments for use in measuring this type of radiation have been developed for commercial production.

The atoms of radon progeny form in the air due to decay of radon (emanations). The experimental data on diffusion coefficient of emanation shows the value in the range of 0.08–0.12 cm^2/s for radon, 0.112–0.125 for actinon, and 0.085–0.103 for thoron. According to different authors, diffusion coefficient of radon

Nanoparticles in Humans: Experiments, Methods, and Strategies
Lev S. Ruzer

ISBN 978-981-4463-16-4 (Hardcover), 978-981-4463-17-1 (eBook)
www.panstanford.com

Table 3.1 Three groups of charged radon progeny with different electrical mobility, k_{el}

	k_{el1}	k_{el2}	k_{el3}
Air–nitrogen	1.80 ± 0.20	0.85 ± 0.15	0.55 ± 0.1
Oxygen	1.90 ± 0.22	0.90 ± 0.20	0.50 ± 0.14
CO_2	1.50 ± 0.23	0.75 ± 0.15	0.50 ± 0.14
Ar	1.65 ± 0.20	0.82 ± 0.15	0.40 ± 0.10
He	3		

progeny unattached activity is in the range of 0.045–0.068 cm^2/s, i.e., approximately two times less than for emanations. Such big difference suggested that unattached activity consists not of atoms but of molecules complex, which forms as a result of chemical or physical interaction between radioactive atoms and molecules of different gases, which was confirmed by different experiments.

In an experiment with diffusion batteries, Madelaine (1966) showed that in the clear (no dust) air, diffusion coefficient of unattached activity decreased during "age" and after 1 h became equal to 0.028 cm^2/s. The author suggested that the effect can be explained by the attachment of unattached activity to molecules of H_2O, O_2, and other admixtures.

Ferrin et al. (1966) found three groups of charged radon progeny with different electrical mobility, k_{el}, as shown in Table 3.1.

Studies suggested that the time of life of primary atoms is proximally 0.8 sec and that primary atoms attach to gas molecules or admixture.

Similar results were presented in Bricard et al. (1966), where researchers found that unattached activity consists of five groups with electrical mobility of 2.10 ± 0.20; 1.35 ± 0.15; 0.88 ± 0.10; 0.58 ± 0.07; 0.43 ± 0.03 ($cm^2/s.v$).

Fontan et al. (1968) studied the "aging" of diffusion coefficient of radon and thoron unattached activity number by means of diffusion batteries. It was found that neutral radioactive atoms of ThB by the age of 20 sec have diffusion coefficient of 0.02 cm^2/s and after 10 min 0.01 cm^2/s, and then decreasing became smaller.

Hence, the range of diffusion coefficient of unattached fraction of radon progeny is in the range of 0.10–0.01 (Table 3.2).

Table 3.2 Range of diffusion coefficient of unattached fraction of radon progeny

	D (range) (cm^2/s)	Method
Madelaine, 1966	0.5–0.28	Diffusion
Ferrin et al., 1966	0.05–0.01	Electrostatic
Bricard et al., 1966	0.06–0.01	Electrostatic
Fontain et al., 1968	0.09–0.01	Diffusion

3.1.1 *The Attachment of Atoms of Radon Progeny to Non-Radioactive Aerosols*

Theory of processes of the attachment of radon progeny atoms to non-radioactive aerosols is presented in Knutson (1988) and Polev (1967).

In time-changing concentration of unattached activity is described by the following equation:

$$(dn_i/dt) = \lambda_{I-1}n_{I-1} - \lambda_I n_I - \lambda_I n_I \int K(r)N(r)dr, \tag{3.1}$$

where I is the number of progeny, n_{I} is the concentration of I-th product, λ_{I} the decay constant of the I-th product, $N(r)dr$ the aerosol particle concentration in the range r–$r+dr$, and $K(r)$ the coagulation constant of unattached activity to aerosols particles with a radius r. The integral $\int K(r)N(r)dr$ on whole spectrum of aerosol sizes (5×10^{-7} - 2×10^{-3} cm) determines the speed of coagulation of unattached activity with aerosol. The time by which the number of unattached atoms diminished two times (attached half-time) is $T_{\mathrm{p}} = \ln 2/\lambda_{\mathrm{p}}$.

In time-changing concentration $N(r)$ with radius r, and attached I product is described by the following equation:

$$(dN_i/dt) = K(r)N(r)_I n_I + \lambda_{I-1}N_{I-1}(r) - \lambda_I N_I(r) \tag{3.2}$$

Coagulation constant $K(r)$ is determined by collisions of unattached activity with aerosols particles due to Brown diffusion and electrostatic interaction in case charged particles. For aerosols with the size $r > 10^{-5}$ cm coagulation due to Brown diffusion is described by diffusion equations. In this case, the coagulation constant is $K(r) = 4\pi Dr$, where D is the diffusion coefficient of unattached activity and r the aerosol particle radius. In this equation the aerosol particle itself implies to be immobile relatively to the unattached activity. Its movement can be described by means of an addition of aerosol diffusion coefficient to unattached activity diffusion coefficient

For aerosols with $r < 10^{-7}$ cm, coagulation takes place in gas kinetic manner according to the following formula: $K(r) = \pi v r^2$, where $v = \sqrt{(8kT)/\pi}$, v is the average gas kinetic velocity of unattached activity under absolute temperature T, and m the mass of the particles.

For intermediate range of sizes formula is

$$K(r) = \pi v r^2[(r + \lambda)/(r + \lambda + vr^2/4D), \quad (3.3)$$

where λ is free path of the unattached activity.

In case of electrically charged atoms of radon progeny, their attachment to neutral particle will increase the aerosol particles' attachment velocity. Taking into account electrostatic attachment, coagulation constant $K'(r)$ can be obtained by changing geometric particle radius on action radius r' according to the following:

$$\bar{V} = (ek_{\text{el}})/rr'(r/r' - r'/r)^2, \quad (3.4)$$

where e is the electron charge, k_{el} the electrical mobility of unattached activity, and $\bar{V}$ the average gas kinetic velocity of unattached activity.

Table 3.3 presents the action radius for the assessment of the dependence of electrostatic attachment on the particle radius.

As we can see from Table 3.3, electrostatic attachment plays a substantial role only for particles size of $r < 1 \times 10^{-5}$ cm.

Table 3.3 Action radius for the assessment of the dependence of electrostatic attachment from particle radius

r (cm)	r'/r
2×10^{-7}	7.9
5×10^{-7}	4.4
1×10^{-6}	2.9
2×10^{-6}	2.0
5×10^{-6}	1.4
1×10^{-5}	1.0

RaA, the first daughter product, is formed by Rn-222 decay in the form of single atoms, which diffuse rapidly through the air. These atoms may attach themselves very rapidly to the molecules of water vapor, or other polar impurities in the air, to form unattached activity to diffuse rapidly through air. Apart from removal by ventilation, they are subject to deposition in walls and other surfaces or to attachment to condensation nuclei and dust particles. When the RaA and the subsequent daughter come into contact with any surface, they attach themselves to it very firmly, consisting of—as they do—elements (polonium, bismuth, and lead) that all are solid at room temperature. The rate of deposition on uncharged surfaces is controlled by the rate of diffusion to the surface rather than upon the chemical nature of the surface and it is probable that every unattached cluster diffusing to the surface is retained there.

Under atmospheric conditions, some of these clusters will attach themselves to typically small particles, which are inevitably present in the air. These airborne particles range from condensation nuclei of a few hundredths of microns in radius to others of a few microns in size. Table 3.4 presents the distribution of radioactivity against particle-size range for typical atmospheric conditions.

According to Chamberlain and Dyson (1956), the unattached activity deposition is 800 and 600 time higher in cylindrical tubes and in model of larynx and trachea, respectively, than that for aerosols.

In this connection, it was postulated that in case of high unattached concentration, the additional irradiation of the upper lung will be possible.

Table 3.4 Distribution of radioactivity against particle-size range for typical atmospheric conditions

Particle size	% of total radioactivity (microns)
<005	5
0.005–0.015	25
0.015–0.025	50
0.025–0.035	10
0.035 to >0.035	10

In 1959, the ICRP established the new maximum permissible concentration (MPC) for radon:

$$\text{MPC} = 3 \times 10^{-9}/(1 + 1000\, f_\text{A})\text{Ci/l}, \tag{3.5}$$

where f_A is part of the equilibrium of RaA unattached activity in the air, which equals approximately 0.1 for filtrated atmospheric air.

3.1.2 *Equilibrium Conditions between Unattached Activity, Aerosols, and Surface Activity*

Consider the buildup of RaA in air from a constant Rn-222 source concentration (a_0):

$(n_\text{a})_\text{f}$ unattached activity RaA concentration

$(n_\text{a})_\text{p}$ aerosol concentration

λ_A RaA decay constant

λ_p decay constant of adsorption of unattached activity to aerosol particles

λ_s effective rate constant for depletion by surface adsorption of unattached activity

Then

$$[d(n_\text{a})_\text{f}/dt] = a_0 - (\lambda_\text{s} + \lambda_\text{A} + \lambda_\text{p})(n_\text{a})_\text{f} \tag{3.6}$$

$$\text{i.e.,} \quad (n_\text{a})_\text{f} = (a_0)/(\lambda_\text{s} + \lambda_\text{A} + \lambda_\text{p})[1 - \exp[-(\lambda_\text{s} + \lambda_\text{A} + \lambda_\text{p})t], \tag{3.7}$$

and at equilibrium,

$$(n_\text{a})_\text{f} = (a_0)/(\lambda_\text{s} + \lambda_\text{A} + \lambda_\text{p}). \tag{3.8}$$

For total material airborne (i.e., aerosols plus unattached activity),

$$(n_\text{a})_\text{e} = (a_0)/(\lambda_\text{s} + \lambda_\text{A}) \tag{3.9}$$

$$\text{i.e.,}\ (a_\text{A})_\text{e} = a_0\lambda_\text{A}/(\lambda_\text{s} + \lambda_\text{A}). \tag{3.10}$$

Further if we consider the total amounts of RaB and RaC airborne, and for each material we write $\lambda^1 = (\lambda_\text{s} + \lambda)$ (noting that

(λ_s may be different for each daughter) we have in equilibrium:

$$(a_A)_e = a_0\lambda_A/\lambda_A^1 \tag{3.11}$$

$$(a_B)_e = (a_0\lambda_A/\lambda_A^1)(\lambda_B/\lambda_B^1) \tag{3.12}$$

$$(a_C)_e = (a_0\lambda_A/\lambda_A^1)(\lambda_B/\lambda_B^1)(\lambda_C/\lambda_C^1) \tag{3.13}$$

Taking into account once again, the form of airborne material and neglecting the deposition of aerosols, the relevant built-up of aerosols carried activity is governed by

$$[d(n_a)_p/dt] = \lambda_p(n_a)_f - \lambda_A(n_A)_P \tag{3.14}$$

and at final equilibrium,

$$[(n_a)_p]\text{ equil} = (\lambda_p/\lambda_A)[(n_a)_f]\text{ equil}, \tag{3.15}$$

$$\text{i.e., } [(n_a)_p]\text{ equil} = (\lambda_p/\lambda_A)a_0/(\lambda_s + \lambda_A + \lambda_p). \tag{3.16}$$

Thus, in equilibrium conditions, the unattached fraction will be

$$f = [(n_a)_f\text{ equil}]/\{[(n_a)_f]\text{ equil} + [(n_a)_p]\text{ equil}\} \tag{3.17}$$

$$\text{i.e., } f = 1/[1 + (\lambda_p/\lambda_A)] = \lambda_A/(\lambda_A + \lambda_p). \tag{3.18}$$

The unattached fraction f is important for assessing the inhalation hazard from daughter products. The corresponding values of f for both RaA and RaB are shown in Table 3.5 derived from rate-

Table 3.5 Values of f for RaA and RaB

			Unattached fraction $f = \lambda/(\lambda + \lambda_p)$	
Particle conc. (cm^{-3})	λ_p	$1/\lambda_p$	RaA	RaC
10^2	4.4×10^{-6}	2.4×10^5	1.00	0.99
10^3	4.4×10^{-5}	2.4×10^4	0.99	0.93
10^4	4.4×10^{-4}	2.4×10^3	0.90	0.57
5×10^4	2.2×10^{-3}	1.2×10^3	0.63	0.22
10^5	4.4×10^{-3}	2.4×10^2	0.46	0.12
10^6	4.4×10^{-2}	2.4	0.09	0.01
10^7	4.4×10^{-1}	0.24	0.01	0.00

adsorption constants calculated for a range of concentrations of particles of 0.2 μm mean diameter.

3.1.3 *Size (Diffusion Coefficient) Distribution of the Unattached Activity*

The tests (Holub and Knutson, 1987) of the newly developed graded wire screen method for measuring the size and amount of "unattached" radon progeny were done as part of the Radon-Aerosol Workshop (OECD and CEC) held in March 1987 at the Australian Radiation Laboratory. Comparisons were made between different sets of graded wire screens, and between the screen and conventional diffusion batteries, under conditions of high and of low aerosol concentration. Also, two mathematical methods for de-convoluting the data were compared. Results from different graded screen configurations agreed well as to size of the 'unattached' progeny; modal diameters varied from about 0.7 to 1.5 nm, i.e., from atomic dimensions to dimensions of a cluster of molecules. There were differences of about a factor of two in the measured amount, but this appears to be a function of sampling location rather than screen configuration. Diffusion battery results for the 'unattached' progeny did not agree with the screen results, particularly as to size. For attached radon progeny, the graded screen results were surprisingly consistent with results from diffusion batteries. Also, the two deconvolution methods yielded substantially the same results when applied to the screen data.

To measure the unattached fraction of radon progeny, a new type of portable, low-cost, reusable integrating monitor with etched track detector (CR-39) was developed. This monitor simultaneously gives the average equilibrium-equivalent concentrations of unattached (222)Rn progeny (EEC(Rn)(u)), attached (222)Rn progeny (EEC(Rn)(a)) and also (220)Rn progeny (EEC(Tn)). It was calculated, according to the detection efficiencies that were derived by the Monte Carlo method, that the lower detection limits for EEC(Rn)(u), EEC(Rn)(a) and EEC(Tn) are 0.03 Bq m^{-3}, 0.12 Bq m^{-3}, and 0.07 Bq m^{-3}, respectively, for 24 h integrating sampling at a flow rate of 2.92 l min^{-1}. The validity of the new monitor was confirmed through a series of intercomparison experiments.

3.1.4 *A Nuclear Mass Spectrometer for Studying Radon Progeny Cluster*

Gong et al. (1996) measured the cluster formation of radon progeny ^{218}Po in gaseous H_2O and H_2O–SO_2 mass spectrometer and the low detection efficiency. This NMS combines the mass-separation ability of a mass spectrometer and the low detection limit of a surface barrier detector for alpha particles and enables the detection of individual radon progeny cluster ions of defined mass at the molecular level. Clusters in the form of $^{218}Po{+}(H_2O)_n$ were experimentally observed for ^{218}Po at a relative humidity of 0.1%. The number *n* ranged from 1 to 7 with 4 being the most abundant peak under these conditions. No charged cluster of ^{218}Po was detected when relative humidity was 90%, possibly due to neutralization process. On addition of SO_2 at a low relative humidity $^{218}Po{+}(H_2O)_n(H_2SO_4)_m$, clusters were experimentally detected for the first time.

For a system in this study with *n* from 0 to 4 and *m* from 0 to 3, the maximum distribution occurs at a radius of about 3.65 Å or a mobility of about 2.00 $cm^2/s.v.$ These maximum clusters correspond to a composition of $^{218}Po{+}(H_2SO_4)_1$ or $^{218}Po{+}(H_2O)_2\ (H_2SO_4)_1$.

One such type of instrument was used for measuring the unattached activity in mines (Kartashev, 1966, 1967)—wire screen method (instrument "RB–alpha").

Aerosol radiometer type "RB–alpha" was intended for the measurement of the concentration of alpha-active aerosols of radon (thoron) progeny in atmosphere of mines and other industrial environments. The instrument also measured the concentration of unattached activity of RaA.

In this instrument, the membrane diffusion screen was used as a selective sampler of the unattached activity of RaA. The sampler consists of a copper foil with thickness of 4.5×10^{-3} cm with numbers of cylindrical apertures of 4.9×10^{-3} per cm^2 with radius of 3.7×10^{-3} cm and area of 0.43×10^{-4} cm^2.

The deposition coefficient θ of the unattached activity with the diffusion coefficient of 0.054 cm^2s^{-1} was calculated according to the formulas given in Gormley et al. (1949). For the velocity of penetration through diffusion battery 250 cm/s it was equal to 0.33.

Effectiveness of registration of alpha particles from battery aperture was $\varepsilon = \chi c$, where c is a constant of calibration of detector and χ the geometric coefficient of departure of radiation from the channels of diffusion battery (wire screen); $\varepsilon = 0.152$; $\chi = 0.475$.

The review of the reliability of different methods for measuring the unattached activity, including some theoretical consideration, is provided in Polev (1967).

Most commonly used methods for measuring the unattached fraction are based on their small size and therefore high diffusion coefficient. It should be mentioned, however, that the real deposition coefficient of the unattached activity on the walls of a cylindrical tube, the wires of the screen and the channels of walls of diffusion batteries can have different values from 0% to 100%.

For the assessment of the reliability of instrumentation in this case as for other measurement techniques, the standard and calibration technique should be developed. This technique should provide an opportunity for generating with good stability and measurement with great accuracy the unattached fraction of radon decay products in all range of its value, including close to 0% and 100%. Such standard and calibration technique was developed in the frames of the Special State Standard for the Volumetric Activity of Radioactive Aerosols in the former USSR (Antipin et al., 1980).

3.2 Correlation between the Unattached Activity of Radon Decay Products and Aerosol Concentration

Aerosol concentration can be expressed in several ways, such as particle number, as particle surface area, and a particle volume (mass), depending upon on the aerosol properties of interest. The particle surface area concentration (expressed in units of cm^2/cm^3 or cm^{-1}) is an important parameter in the study of the interaction of radon decay products with available aerosols. The aerosol surface also plays a role in the behavior of gas-phase species indoors, such as polycyclic aromatic hydrocarbons, as it is a side for sorption and desorption of these species (Yamasaki et al., 1982; Pistikopoulos et al., 1990).

Light scattering is one of the main physical effects on which instruments for measuring small aerosol concentrations are based. It is widely used, for example, in the measurement of particle number concentrations through the use of a condensation nuclei counter or in measuring the size distribution of aerosols by means of an optical particle counter. In some cases, such as for optical particle counters, there are lower limits to the sizes of particles detected, typically in the vicinity of 0.1 μm.

Since the distribution of the radiation dose in the lung is not uniform but is highly dependent on the proportion of unattached activity compared with that associated with the co-existing aerosol, many studies have been devoted to developing both the theory and techniques for measuring the unattached fraction and to the study both theoretically and experimentally of the correlation between unattached fraction and aerosol concentration. In the past years, the technique based on collection of the airborne activity on wire mesh screens has become most commonly used method for estimating the unattached fraction of radon decay products.

The theoretical basis for using high mobility of the unattached activity concentration (AAC) in measurement of diffusion deposition was laid down in Gormley et al. (1949).

The main expression for the "passage" (the ratio of the average concentrations of monodispersed aerosols on the exit and enter of the cylindrical tube) due to diffusion deposition was presented in the following form:

$$k = \begin{cases} 0.8191e^{-7.314h} + 0.0975e^{-44.6h} + 0.0325e^{-114h}, & h > 0.0156 \quad (3.19) \\ 1 - 4.07h^{2/3} + 2.4h + 0.446h^{2/3}, & h < 0.0156 \end{cases}$$

$$(3.20)$$

where k is a passage, $h = Dl/2Q$, l the length of the tube, Q the volume aerosol passing rate, and D the diffusion coefficient of aerosol particles.

For practical purposes, it is necessary to determine conditions for applying Eqs. 3.19 and 3.20 in all range of the AAC sizes, because it was derived on the basis of simplified assumptions. It is also necessary to study the possibility of using the diffusion method for the determination of polydispersed aerosol parameters.

Because of the sharp decrease in diffusion deposition with particle size, a set of parallel channels (diffusion batteries) is practically used for AAC aerosol measurement, which allows to automatically decrease the volume rate to the necessary degree. The biggest battery in a few studies had 3700 cylindrical tubes (m = 3700) and length l = 20 cm, i.e., the summary length of the channels mL, which is a parameter of the deposition capability, was 74,000. This was not enough for the study of AAC in all range of sizes of the aerosol particles. In addition, due to the battery's 20 cm diameter, it was practically impossible to provide for laminar flow in the diffuser, which connects the battery with communications.

Below are the results of experiments in laboratory conditions carried out by Dokukina et al. (1974). These conditions allow changing the aerosol concentration in broad limits with simultaneously measuring both the radon decay products unattached concentration and aerosol concentration.

In this study, the correlation between unattached fraction of ^{218}Po and aerosols was studied in a 2 m^3 calibration chamber. The chamber has an inlet for introducing Rn and aerosols and an outlet for collecting samples of radon decay products and measuring aerosol concentration. In separate experiments for each aerosol size, seven different sizes of monodispersed latex aerosol, ranging from 0.3 to 2.1 μm, were generated and injected into the chamber. Their concentration was measured using aerosol counter, type AZ-5, which operates on the basis of light scattering. This instrument was a standard aerosol counter in widespread use in the former Soviet Union.

Measurement of the ^{218}Po unattached activity was done using a rectangular diffusion battery followed by backing filter. An open-face filter operated in parallel to the diffusion battery sampled the total airborne ^{218}Po activity. A single-channel alpha particle spectrometer was used to count ^{218}Po alpha particles. This device consisted of a Cs (Tl) scintillator coupled to a photomultiplier tube, which, along with the appropriate electronics, identified the alpha particles from decay of ^{218}Po [24]. The diffusion battery consisted of a flat brass disc 2.3 mm thick with 117 rectangular apertures, each 0.18 mm wide and 5 mm high (Fig. 3.1).

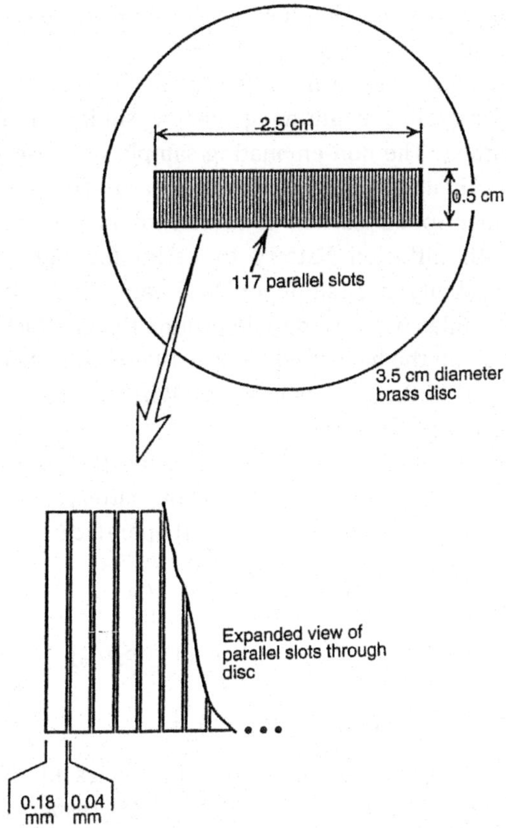

Figure 3.1 Disc diffusion battery with 117 rectangular channels. Each channel measures 0.18 mm × 5 mm. The disc has a thickness of 2.3 mm. The expanded view shows a portion of the parallel slots in more detail. Copyright (2012). From *Aerosols Handbook: Measurement, Dosimetry, and Health Effects*, Second Edition, edited by Lev S. Ruzer and Naomi H. Harley. Reproduced by permission of Taylor and Francis Group, LLC, a division of Informa plc.

The 3.5 cm diameter of the diffusion battery disc was the same as the diameter of the standard filter used to collect the aerosol. The filter samplers were specially designed filters (filter type LFS) used for alpha spectroscopy measurements.

A non-emanating sample of ^{226}Ra, also deposited on a 3.5 cm disc, was used to calibrate the efficiency of the detector for ^{218}Po deposited on or in the channels of the diffusion battery and for activity deposited on the filter.

For the former case, a mask was built for the non-emanating sample to provide a counting geometry similar to that of the diffusion battery. The non-emanating sample was also used to set up the discriminator windows for the alpha spectrometer.

As we mentioned earlier, it is critical in the measurement provided with diffusion battery to determine the efficiency of unattached activity deposition on the walls of the battery. The following formulas were used to determine the unattached fraction of ^{218}Po based on the measured alpha activities. The same formulas should be used in the studies based on wire mesh screen or other types of measurement techniques.

If N_i is the detected ^{218}Po activity for the three collection surfaces, where i = db for the diffusion battery; i = bf for the backing filter and i = of for the (parallel) open-face filter, then

$$N_{\text{db}} = e_1 e_3 A_\text{u} + e_2 e_4 A_\text{a} \tag{3.21}$$

$$N_{\text{bf}} = e[(1 - e_1)A_\text{u} + (1 - e_2)A_\text{a}] \tag{3.22}$$

$$N_{\text{of}} = e(A_\text{u} + A_\text{a}) = eA_\text{t}, \tag{3.23}$$

where e_1 and e_2 are the collection efficiencies of the diffusion battery for the unattached and attached ^{218}Po, respectively; e_3 and e_4 are the detection efficiencies for the unattached and attached ^{218}Po deposited on/in the diffusion battery, respectively; e is the detection efficiency for ^{218}Po alpha activity collected on the filter; and A_u, A_a, and A_t are the airborne activity concentrations of the unattached, attached, and total ^{218}Po activity, respectively. The unattached fraction, f, of ^{218}Po is defined as

$$f = A_\text{u}/A_\text{t}. \tag{3.24}$$

The detection efficiency for the ^{218}Po activity collected on the filters, denoted as e in Eqs. 3.22 and 3.23 was determined using the non-emanating radium source noted earlier, which had the same source-detector geometry as activity on the filters. Because this calibration source is non-emanating, the ^{222}Rn and its short-lived decay products are in complete radioactive equilibrium with the ^{226}Ra parent; thus the detection efficiency for the ^{218}Po alpha particles can be easily measured. In the case of the diffusion battery, the parameters of the battery were originally calculated using formulas for diffusion deposition in rectangular channels [26]. The size of the channels was selected to achieve a collection efficiency for the unattached fraction ^{218}Po of nearly 100%. The battery and the measurement technique itself were then calibrated experimentally using the chamber with 100% of the ^{218}Po unattached (achieved by near-zero aerosol concentration) and a zero level of unattached ^{218}Po, corresponding to an aerosol concentration of $> 10^6$ particles cm^{-3}. These two cases provided the means for determining the collection and detection efficiencies based on Eqs. 3.21–3.23, as follows:

At 100% unattached $A_t \sim A_u$; so $N_{of} = eA_u$ from Eq. 3.23, or regarding, $A_u = N_{of}/e$. Then from Eq. 3.22,

$$N_{bf} = e(1 - e_1)A_u = (1 - e_1)N_{of} \tag{3.25}$$

and

$$e_1 = 1 - N_{bf}/N_{of}. \tag{3.26}$$

The detection efficiency for the unattached ^{218}Po deposited on the diffusion battery can be found from Eqs. 3.21 and 3.23:

$$e_3 = eN_{db}/e_1 N_{of} \tag{3.27}$$

Similarly, at 100% attached, $A_t = A_a$, so $A_a = N_{of}/e$. Then from Eq. 3.22,

$$N_{bf} = e(1 - e_2)A_a = (1 - e_2)N_{of} \tag{3.28}$$

and

$$e_2 = 1 - N_{bf}/N_{of}. \tag{3.29}$$

The detection efficiency for the unattached ^{218}Po deposited on the diffusion battery is

$$e_4 = eN_{db}/e_2 N_{of}. \tag{3.30}$$

Chamber calibration experiments were conducted using both monodisperse aerosols and known mixtures of different aerosol sizes to determine the operating parameters of the diffusion battery. Based on these experiments the deposition and detection efficiency parameters of the diffusion battery are: $e_1 = 0.95$; $e_2 = 0.24$ (this depends on the particle size distribution; the value used here in an average of all calibration aerosol sizes); $e_3 = 0.33$ and $e_4 = 0.24$. The difference in detection efficiency is due to difference in deposition location of the unattached and attached ^{218}Po within diffusion battery aperture.

Based on Eqs. 3.24 and combining Eqs. 3.21 and 3.22, a formula for the unattached fraction of ^{218}Po in terms of measured quantities can be derived:

$$f = A_u e / N_{of}$$
$$= [eN_{db}(1 - e_2) - e_2 e_4 N_{bf}] / N_{of}[e_1 e_3 (1 - e_2) - e_2 e_4 (1 - e_1)] \quad (3.31)$$

This formula applies generally to any similar system. This approach can be used, for example, with methods designed to increase the collection of low concentration of radioactive aerosols, by using higher flow rates and/or modified diffusion batteries, as long as appropriate calibration procedures can be used to provide the efficiency parameters in Eqs. 3.29.

Summary of results of this approach are presented in Fig. 3.2, which shows the unattached concentration of ^{218}Po relative to particle surface area concentration, based on calibration measurements made with monodispersed latex aerosols of different sizes and concentrations [27].

In each case, the measured aerosol concentration was converted to the aerosol surface area concentration. These results suggest that for aerosols in the sizes range covered by this calibration, from 0.3 to 2.1 μm in diameter, the particle surface area concentration, s in the corresponding range from 10^{-5} to 0.3 cm^{-1} is related to the unattached fraction of ^{218}Po, f. This is the basis for the approach proposed here for measuring small concentration of aerosols (Ruzer, 1984).

The calibration procedure used here relies upon monodisperse spherical particles, from which surface area can be directly calculated. In practice, an "equivalent surface area" should be used, which is surface area of a spherical aerosol having the same diffusion deposition property as the real aerosol. Under actual measurement conditions (e.g., in a building or in a mine), the only measurements

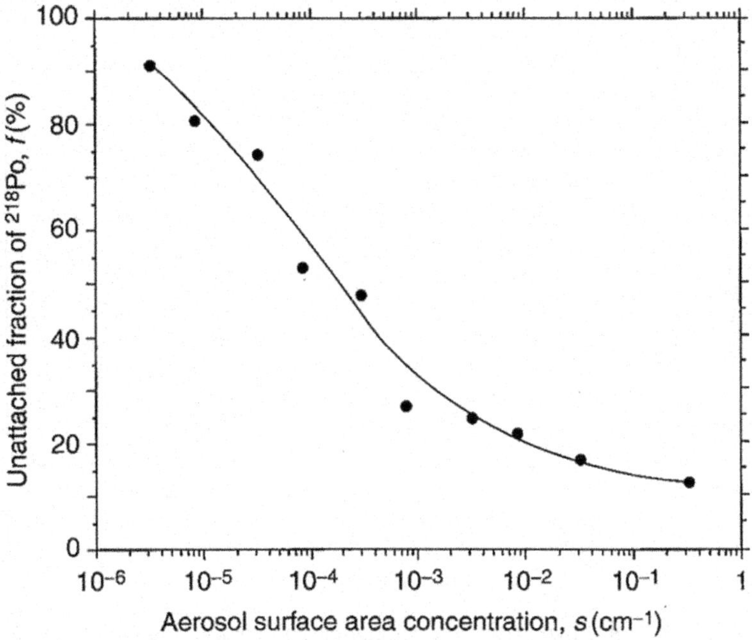

Figure 3.2 Measures ^{218}Po unattached fraction plotted against particle surface area concentration based on the calibration experiments with the rectangular diffusion battery. The line is to guide the eye. Copyright (2012). From *Aerosols Handbook: Measurement, Dosimetry, and Health Effects*, Second Edition, edited by Lev S. Ruzer and Naomi H. Harley. Reproduced by permission of Taylor and Francis Group, LLC, a division of Informa plc.

necessary to determine the unattached fraction and to infer the average aerosol surface area are those described above—a diffusion battery followed by a backing filter and an open face filter operated in parallel. The alpha activity from ^{218}Po on each of these three collectors is then measured and used with appropriate calibration factors to yield the unattached fraction.

The curves in Fig. 3.2 can be used for calibration purposes. For example, for spherical particles with diameter of 0.1 μm and 1.0 μm and concentration of 10^5 cm^{-3}, the particle surface area concentration is 3×10^{-5} cm^{-1} and 3×10^{-3} cm^{-1}, respectively. The corresponding unattached fractions of ^{218}Po are 70% and 25%, respectively.

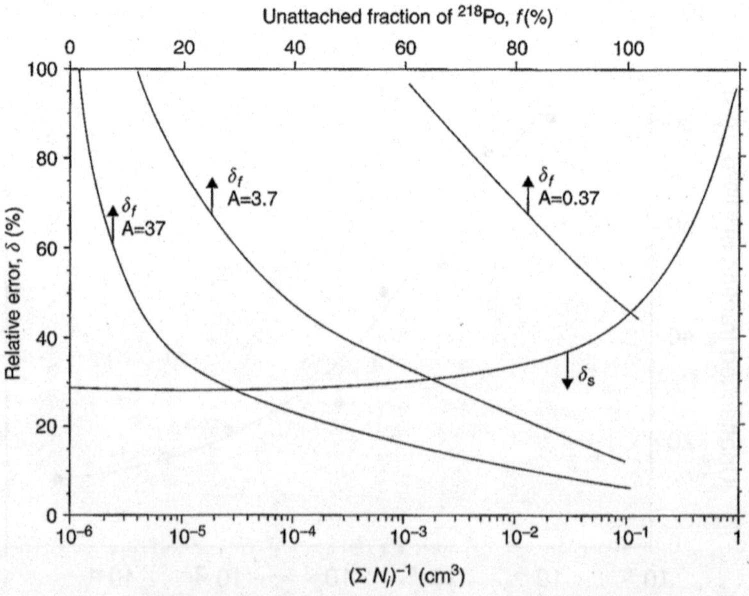

Figure 3.3 Relative errors (in estimating Po activity). Copyright (2012). From *Aerosols Handbook: Measurement, Dosimetry, and Health Effects*, Second Edition, edited by Lev S. Ruzer and Naomi H. Harley. Reproduced by permission of Taylor and Francis Group, LLC, a division of Informa plc.

Figure 3.3 shows calculated errors in measurements of both s and f. Errors for f were calculated for three different total activity concentrations of ^{218}Po.

The estimated error for the area of particles of any size, i, is shown as a function of $(1/N_i)$, where N_i is the concentration of particles of the i-th size range. Combining the results shown in Figs. 3.2 and 3.3 allows the estimation of the lower detection limit on aerosol concentration afforded by this approach. From Fig. 3.2, the largest unattached fraction measurement achieved in the calibration chamber, 92%, corresponds to the aerosol concentration of 3×10^{-6} cm^{-1}. In terms of particle number concentration, the limits, which depend upon particle size, are from 20 (at 2.1 μm particle diameter) to 1000 particles cm^{-3} (at 0.3 μm particle diameter). For these concentrations, relative errors range from 30% to 40% as shown in Fig. 3.3.

Quantitative comparison of results of the experiments described here with those previously reported presents some difficulties because most of the previously reported measurements were conducted in the laboratory conditions that yielded a wide range of unattached fraction for similar aerosol conditions. These studies did not directly investigate the problem of measurement and calibration across a broad range of aerosol and radon decay products concentrations, particularly in the case of low aerosol concentration and the concomitant high fraction of unattached radon progeny.

An examination of Figs. 3.2 and 3.3 provides an indication of the applicability of the proposed method. Two factors are important: (1) The unattached fraction of ^{218}Po should be at least 15–20% or higher to provide sensitivity to changes in particle surface area concentration, and (2) the amount of ^{218}Po collected should be enough to achieve the desired statistical accuracy. As a practical matter, these conditions exist in many underground mining situations and in some residual environments.

3.3 Measurements of Other Radon Decay Product Unattached Activity Concentration

In the most of the studies, only ^{218}Po unattached fraction concentration measurements were provided. This based on that both from theoretical consideration and some experimental results the concentrations of the unattached ^{214}Bi and ^{214}Pb are much smaller than for that for unattached ^{218}Po. This is true in terms of concentration.

However, from the point of view of the contribution to the dose, the unattached activity of ^{214}Bi and ^{214}Pb should not be ignored according to the formula for Potential Alpha Energy Concentration (PAEC), which is equally true both for attached and unattached activity:

$$\mathrm{PAEC} = 1.05q_a + 5.16q_b + 3.80q_c \tag{3.32}$$

One of the examples of such study is presented in Kojima and Abe (1988).

Continual and simultaneous measurements of unattached radon daughters (RaA, RaB, RaC) and the total radon daughters were performed in a house under normal living conditions, which include ordinary living habits, the style of house construction, and the normal natural ventilation rate in Japan. The hourly concentrations of three radon daughters were obtain separately and simultaneously with a radon daughter monitor, which has air filtration and gross alpha counting systems. The instrument was automatically operated (and maintenance-free) over a period of two months.

The unattached atoms of radon daughters were measured with another radon daughter monitor with the wire screens substituting for the filter. From the measurements for seven months (1986–1987), it can be stated that

1. the concentration of RaA is the most predominant of these daughters, and the unattached RaB is always detectable;
2. the median value of the unattached fraction, indicated by potential alpha energy f_p, is around 0.04, and RaB makes a contribution of more than 30% to the overall f_p; and
3. the data for the unattached fraction show a typical diurnal variation, having a low level in intervals of 7 to 9 and 20 to 22 local hours. This corresponds to aerosol generation from the use of gas ranges in the house.

The collection of the unattached radon daughters was done by a wire screen of 500 mesh with a roll shape 10 m long and 60 mm wide. Using this apparatus, the hourly data for a continual five days were obtained. Since the counting efficiency of the wire screen is not the same as that of the membrane filter due to attachment of the some of the unattached daughters to the back of the screen, the authors used special procedure to obtain the correction factor, i.e., using two types of technique—for unattached and attached measurements. This correction factor was 0.790.

As some of unattached atoms may adhere to the monitor's sampling head during the sampling, which will decrease unattached radon daughters collected on the wire screen, another correction factor was introduced using other type of experiments. This factor was 0.820 (normalized to the result of the filter sampler) at the flow rate of $35\,\mathrm{l{\cdot}m^{-1}}$. The concentration of RaA and RaB was estimated to be about 2 and 0.3 Bq·m^{-3}, respectively, with a standard deviation of 50%.

Field measurements were conducted in a detached two-storied concrete house under ordinary living conditions in Japan. In the house, the mechanical ventilation system was not set. Frequency of door and window opening increased during the hot summer months. In cold months, the rooms in the house were heated by oil heaters. The ventilation rate was found to be 0.4 to 0.8 per hour with closed windows. The apparatus were set in a living room at the ground floor of the house. The total radon daughters were measured continuously without a pause, and unattached radon daughters were measured for about 10 days in a month. Other parameters, such as aerosol particles, were measured only occasionally.

In these measurements, the unattached RaA had the highest concentration and RaB the second highest. The unattached RaC was extremely low and therefore can be ignored if the aerosol concentration is in a range between 3×10^3 and 2×10^4 cm^{-3}.

However, unattached RaB cannot be ignored because its concentration is 10–20% of that unattached RaA.

The authors considered that the difference in concentration found between unattached RaB and unattached RaC would be due to the recoil effect of alpha decay of attached RaA which will produce some unattached RaB.

3.4 The Effect of Recoil Nuclei Being Knocked Off Aerosol Particles Unattached Concentration of Radon Decay Products (Kolerski et al., 1973)

At present, the common opinion is that radon atoms do not deposit on aerosol particles and consequently the unattached daughters of the first decay product are developed only by decay of the atoms of Rn. However, the atoms of the second, third, and so forth daughter products can be developed by the two ways: from the unattached fraction of the previous daughter products by its decay; from attached fraction to aerosol particle atoms of the previous product, which by its decay recoiled from the aerosol particles due to the "knocking off" (recoil) effect.

Taking into account the recoil under radioactive decay, the equation can be written for the change in time in the concentration of unattached activity of radon progeny:

$$dn_i/dt = \lambda_{i-1}n_{i-1} + \alpha_{i-1}\lambda_{i-1}\mathrm{N}_{i-1} - \lambda_{pi}n_i - \lambda_i n_i, \qquad (3.33)$$

where i is the number of the daughter product, n the unattached concentration of the corresponding product, λ the decay constant, α the recoil coefficient (the ratio of numbers of attached atoms of the i-th product, which will recoil under radioactive decay, N_i the concentration of aerosol particles with i-th decay product, λ_{pi} the constant of deposition of the i-th product to the aerosol particles. When the aerosol concentration does not change or changes insignificantly, it is possible to say that λ_{pi} is proportional to the aerosol concentration, i.e.,

$$\lambda_{pi} = k \times N. \qquad (3.34)$$

For the equilibrium situation, i.e., for $dn_i/dt = 0$ and $dN_i/dt = 0$, the expressions for the n_i and N_i will be

$$n_i = (\lambda_{i-1}n_{i-1} + \alpha_{i-1}\lambda_{i-1}N_{i-1})/(\lambda_i + \lambda_{pi}) \qquad (3.35)$$

$$N_i = (\lambda_{pi}n_{i+}(1 - \alpha_{i-1})\lambda_{i-1}N_{i-1})/\lambda_i. \qquad (3.36)$$

The fraction f_i of i-product unattached atoms is

$$f_i = n_i/(n_i + N_i). \qquad (3.37)$$

By substituting for n_i and N_i in Eq. 3.37, their values from Eqs. 3.35 and 3.36, we obtain

$$f_i = [\lambda_i/((\lambda_i + \lambda_{pi})][f_{i-1} + \alpha_{i-1}(1 - f_{i-1})]. \qquad (3.38)$$

Radon is not attached to aerosol particles, and therefore, its unattached atom fraction $f_1 = 1$ and its recoil factor is $\alpha_1 = 0$. By substituting f_2 for f_3, f_3 for f_4, and so forth, we obtain the following general expression for the fraction of i-product of the unattached activity:

$$f_i = f_1[\lambda_k(1 - \alpha_{k-1})/(\lambda_{k+}\lambda_{pk})] + [(\alpha_{j-1}\lambda_j/\lambda_j + \lambda_{pj}) \times (1 - \alpha_{k-1})\lambda_k/(\lambda_k + \lambda_{pk})] + \alpha_{i-1}\lambda_i/\lambda_i + \lambda_{pi} \qquad (3.39)$$

The ejection factor of daughter emanation-product atom aerosol particles, which is produced by recoil in radioactive decay, has not been measured to date. It is obvious that the value of this factor is in the range of 0 to 1. Within the limits, Eq. 3.39 assumes the form

$$f_i = [\lambda_k/(\lambda_k + \lambda_{pk})] \quad \text{for all} \quad \alpha_i = 0 \tag{3.40}$$

and

$$f_i = \lambda_i/(\lambda_i + \lambda_{pi}) \quad \text{for all} \quad \alpha_i = 1. \tag{3.41}$$

The relationship of the fraction of the unattached atoms of radon daughter products from λ_p was calculated from Eqs. 3.40 and 3.41 and represented in the form of curves. In plotting these curves, it was assumed that the permanent attachment of all radon decay products to the aerosol particles is equal to each other. Since $0 < \alpha_i > 1$, the true curves of $f_i = f_i(\lambda_p)$ should be located between the curves of the relationships for $\alpha_i = 0$ and $\alpha_i = 1$. The type and the energy of radiations, which produce the ejection of radioactive atoms from the aerosol particles owing to the recoil effect, determine their position in the main.

It was found that the relative value of the recoil effect contribution to the fraction of the radon daughter's unattached activity increases with a rise in λ_p, i.e., with an increase in the aerosol concentration.

By an analysis of Eq. 3.39, it is possible to suggest the following method for determining experimentally the ejection factor of the unattached decay radon products.

According to Eq. 3.39 and bearing in mind that $f_1 = 1$ and $\alpha_i = 0$, the fraction of the unattached of the first daughter product by radioactive decay can be written as follows:

$$f_2 = \lambda_2/(\lambda_2 + \lambda_p) \tag{3.42}$$

In a similar manner, we can find the unattached atoms for the second products:

$$f_3 = [\lambda_3(\lambda_2 +_+ \lambda_p\alpha_2)]/(\lambda_2 +_+ \lambda_p)(\lambda_{3+} + \lambda_p) \tag{3.43}$$

By eliminating λ_p from Eqs. 3.42 and 3.43, we obtain

$$\alpha_2 = (\lambda_2/\lambda_3 + f_2/(1 - f_2) f_3/f_2 - f_2/(1 - f_2). \tag{3.44}$$

This expression can be used for experimental determination of the ejection factor of the radon decay products atoms from the aerosol particles produced by the recoil effect in the course of the radioactive decay. For this purpose it is necessary to measure the unattached activity fractions f_2 and f_3 of the first and the second decay products, respectively.

In preliminary measurements of the unattached fraction in a chamber where the air was enriched with radon, the following mean values were obtained:

$$f_2(\text{Rae}) = 0.33 \quad \text{and} \quad f_3 = 0.03 \tag{3.45}$$

By using these values in Eq. 3.44 we obtain

$$\alpha_2(\text{Rae}) = 0.4. \tag{3.46}$$

The expression for α_2 (Rae) can be used for evaluation of the contribution to the unattached activity of Rib by the attached Rae atoms, which in the course of the decay were knocked off the aerosol particles. For this purpose, let us rewrite Eq. 3.43 in the following manner:

$$f_3 = \lambda_2\lambda_3/(\lambda_2 + \lambda_p)(\lambda_3 + \lambda_p) + \alpha_2\lambda_3\lambda_p/(\lambda_2 + \lambda_p)(\lambda_3 + \lambda_p) \tag{3.47}$$

3.5 Conclusion

Extensive review of the history of development and utilization of the diffusion batteries as a main tool in measurement of nanometer size particles, including unattached fraction of radon progeny is presented in Knutson (1999).

In Hopke (1992), it was mentioned that the term "unattached fraction" was originally developed for the lung dosimetry, but now some ambiguity exists in its definition between a physical size basis and a dosimetric definition.

Therefore, according to Hopke (1992), we can apply the term "unattached activity" to activity with thermodynamic diameter <2 nm where the atoms of radon progeny are associated with a small number of other molecules. The rest of the radon progeny activity with the size >2 nm can also deposit on the tracheo-bronchial tree.

It should be pointed out, however, that this deposition according to recent studies will be different from uniform because of differences between real structure and unevenness of the inner surface of this part of the lung and that used in modeling.

In reality, as it was shown in Nemmar (2002), the substantial part of the particles in the range of sizes between 5 and 12 nm penetrate tracheo-bronchial tree and through bloodstream deposit on different organs of the body.

The only correct understanding of the role of the unattached fraction in the lung dosimetry can be achieved by using them in experiments on human beings, as it was provided, after approval from special medical committee, in Butterweck et al. (2001).

References

Antipin NI, et al. (1980) *Izmeritel'naya Tekhn* **1**, 5.

Bricard et al. (September 1, 1966a) *CR Acad Sci Paris Ser B* **263**, 761–764.

Bricard et al. (May 9, 1966b) *CR Acad Sci Paris Ser B* **263**, 1315–1317.

Butterweck G, et al. (2001) *Radiation Protection Dosimetry* **94**(3), 247–250.

Chamberlain AC, Dyson ED (1956) *Br J Radiol* **29**, 317–325.

Cooper LA, et al. (1973) *Characteristics of Attached Radon-222 Daughters Under Both Laboratory and Field Conditions*, Battelle, Pacific Northwest Laboratories, Richland, WA.

Dokukina VL, Ruzer LS (1976) *All-Union Institute of Physico-Technical and Radiotechnical Measurements* (VNIIFTRI), Moscow, **30**(60) (in Russian).

Fontan L, et al. (1968).

Fuchs NA (1964) *The Mechanics of Aerosols*. Pergamon, New York.

George AC (1972) *Health Phys* **23**, 390–392.

George AC, Hinchliffe L (1972) *Health Phys* **23**, 791–803.

George AC, et al. (1975) *Am Ind Hyg Assoc J* **36**, 484–490.

Gormley PG, Kennedy M (1949) *Proc R Ir Acad* **52a**, 163.

Gong SL, et al. (1996) *Health Phys* **71**(5), 749–756.

Holub RF, Knutson EO (1987) In *Radon and Its Decay Products: Occurrence, Properties and Health Effects* (Hopke PK, ed.), ACS Symposium Seres 331, American Chemical Society, Washington, DC, pp. 340–356.

Hopke PK (1989) *Environ Int* **15**, 288–308.

Hopke PK (1992) Some thoughts on the "unattached" fraction of radon decay products. *Health Phys* **63**, 209–212.

Kartashev NP (1966) *Atomnaya Energiya* **24**(5), 144.

Kartashev NP (1967) Geophysical Collection, Nuclear Physical Research, No. 6, Ural Branch of the Academy of Sciences of the USSR, Sverdlovsk.

Knutson EO (1988) In *Radon and Its Decay Products in Indoor Air* (Nazaroff WW, Nero AV, ed.), John Wiley, New York, pp. 161–202.

Knutson EO (1999) History of diffusion batteries in aerosol measurement, *Aerosol Sci Technol* **31**, 83–128.

Kojima H, Abe S (1988) Measurement of total and unattached radon daughters in a house, *Radiat Prot Dosim* **24**, 241–244.

Kolerskii SV, Kuznetzov YV, Polev NM, Ruzer LS (1973) *Izmer Tekhn* **10**, 57–58.

Madelaine G (1966) *Tellus*, **18**(2).

Nemmar A, Hoet PH, Vanquickenborne B, Dinsdale D, Thomeer M, Hoylaerts MF, et al. (2002) Passage of inhaled particles into the blood circulation in humans. *Circulation* **105**, 411–414.

Pistikopoulos P, et al. (1990) *Atmos Environ* **24A**, 2573–2584.

Polev NM (1967) Candidate's dissertation, VNIIFTRI, Moscow.

Porstendorfer J (1987) *ACS Symposium Series 331*, Wash., DC; American Chemical Society, pp. 285–300.

Raghavayya M, Jones JH (1974) *Health Phys*, **26**, 417–430.

Reineking A, et al. (1985) *Sci Total Environ* **45**, 261–270.

Ruzer LS (1984) The method of determining the concentration of the gas. Patent No. 234746. Bull. Invent. 28 (in Russian).

Ruzer LS (1993) *Radiation Protection Dosimetry* **46**(2), 127–128.

Zhang L, et al. (2010) *J Radiol Prot* **30**(3), 607–612.

Yamasaki H, et al. (1982) *Environ Sci Technol* **16**, 189–194.

Chapter 4

Method of Direct Measurement of Activity (Dose) in Miners' Lungs

Nomenclature

D: Integral absorbed dose (erg; g-rad)

M: Mass of the lung (g)

D/m: Absorbed dose (rad)

q_i: Radon decay products concentration $i = a, b, c$ $(\mathrm{Bq/m^3})$

v: Rate of inhalation $(\mathrm{m^3 s^{-1}})$

k: Retention coefficient (k)

A_i: Activity in the lung $i = \alpha, \beta, \gamma$ (Bq)

I: Intake (rate of intake) $(\mathrm{Bq\ s^{-1}})$

η_i: Degree of the equilibrium of radon progeny $i = a, b, c$

e: Detection efficiency registration for the decay products

Nanoparticles in Humans: Experiments, Methods, and Strategies
Lev S. Ruzer

ISBN 978-981-4463-16-4 (Hardcover), 978-981-4463-17-1 (eBook)
www.panstanford.com

4.1 Introduction

The determination of the absorbed radiation dose in the lungs of miners due to the inhalation of radon and its decay products can, in principle, be estimated from the air concentration of radon progeny at the work sites, the rate of inhalation and the retention in the lung airways. However, the value of the rate of inhalation is indefinite, since it depends on the physical load (the nature of the work) and varies within broad limits from 10 L/min for the rest to 30–40 L/min for the hard work. The air concentration varies in time and the value of the lung deposition fraction depends on the particle size of the inhaled aerosols and the inhalation rate.

The accurate measurement of the air concentration during exposure is complex. First, the concentration at the same working site is subject to substantial variations. For example, a variation of the intensity of ventilation even for a short time period of time leads to a change in the radon and its progeny concentration of several-fold. Moreover, the content of aerosols directly in the breathing zone may differ substantially from the value measured by an instrument, located in another part of the working area.

Finally, the very concept of the "work place" and "concentration at the work place" are indefinite since miners are at several work places during their work shift, each with different possible concentrations of radon decay products and physical workloads.

For a correct evaluation of the exposure under actual working conditions, we have also taken into account that in some cases miners used respirators for protection of the lung from the aerosol conditions in the mine. All these factors are important for the assessment of the irradiation of the lungs and we will call them "the exposure scenario" or "the working itinerary."

Since practically all measurements of the air concentration of radon progeny at work sites in mines are performed only once or twice a month, there cannot be a precise correspondence between the actual and measured individual (or for group of miners) breathing zone concentrations.

No systematic studies have been made for the assessment of the breathing rate and deposition in lungs for individual or group of miners in real underground conditions. Therefore, it is impossible to calculate the individual exposures correctly.

We present here a method for making direct measurements of the radioactivity in miners' lungs, including the experimental development, the assessment of error, the necessary corrections, and the results of direct measurements of the activity (dose) of miners using portable instruments. The research, i.e., the model and phantom measurements were performed in Moscow (in the former Soviet Union) in the All-Union Institute of Physico-Technical and Radio-Technical Measurements (VNIIFTRI) and Institute of Biophysics (Ministry of Health). The practical application took place in uranium and non-uranium mines in Uzbekistan and Tadjikistan (former USSR). Some aspects of the work have been published, for example (Ruzer et al., 1995). The complete experimental and theoretical details of the method along with the compilation of the results and observed health effects in these mines have not been published before in English.

4.2 Theory of the Method

The basic equations in the most generalized form for the radon series were derived in Ruzer (1958, 1960, 1968). The derivations of the equations are based on the equations described in Bateman (1910) with some appropriate transformations. Bateman's equations for the decay chain transformations were used for the determination of the correlation between the measured air concentration and activity of each decay product on the filter (or lungs).

In order to use these equations for the buildup of activity in the lungs due to filtration, i.e., breathing, we assumed that each member of this chain of decay products supplies the decay products to the lungs at a constant rate $Q_i = q_i vk/\lambda_i$. From a mathematical point of view, the constant rate of supply is equal to the equilibrium between the first and the second member of the chain of radioactive transformation. In this case, the number of the atoms, N, of each decay product in the lungs can be found according to the following equation:

$$N_i = c_1 e^{-\lambda_1 t} + c_2 e^{-\lambda_2 t} + \cdots + c_i e^{-\lambda_i t}, \tag{4.1}$$

where $c_i = N_{1,0} \times \lambda_1 \lambda_2 \ldots \lambda_{i-1}/(\lambda_1 - \lambda_i)\,(\lambda_2 - \lambda_i) \ldots (\lambda_{i-1} - \lambda_i)$ and λ_i is the decay constant of the i-th progeny.

The idea in Ruzer (1958) was to find a correlation between the dose from the alpha radiation of ^{218}Po and ^{214}Po, which cannot be measured directly in the lung and the gamma radiation from ^{214}Pb and ^{214}Bi, which at least theoretically can be measured by external counting. The carcinogenic dose is delivered by the alpha radiation due to its high energy transfer to the cells irradiated.

Due to the gamma emission from the decay products ^{214}Pb and ^{214}Bi and also the relatively high maximum permissible air concentration in comparison with other radioactive aerosols, radon decay products present unique opportunity for the direct measurement of the activity in the lungs.

The final expression for the alpha activity of ^{218}Po and ^{214}Po on the filter (i.e., lungs) is

$$A_\alpha = vk\{q_a[F_a(\theta, t) + F_{a,c}(\theta, t)] + q_b F_{b,c}(\theta, t) + q_c F_{c,c}(\theta, t)\} \tag{4.2}$$

and the corresponding expression for the beta-, and gamma-activity of ^{214}Pb and ^{214}Bi is

$$A_{\beta,\gamma} = vk\{-q_a[F_{a,b}(\theta, t) + F_{a,c}(\theta, t)] + q_b[F_{b,b}(\theta, t) + F_{b,c}(\theta, t) + q_c F_{c,c}(\theta, t)\}. \tag{4.3}$$

The integral absorbed dose to the lung will be

$$D = E_A \int A_a(t)dt + E_{c'} \int A_{c'(t)dt}, \tag{4.4}$$

where E_A and $E_{c'}$ are, respectively, the energies of the alpha particles of ^{218}Po and ^{214}Po.

After series of transformations, Eq. (4.4) can be presented in the form

$$D_a = vk[q_a X_a(\theta) + q_b X_b(\theta) + q_c X_c(\theta)], \tag{4.5}$$

where X_i represents the contribution of each decay products in the absorbed dose.

Equations (4.4) and (4.5) are true for the dose to the whole lung. However, practically measurements were made over the pulmonary region of lung. By comparing Eqs. (4.5) and (4.3), the correlation between the integral absorbed alpha dose to the lung and the gamma activity of ^{214}Pb and ^{214}Bi A_γ, can be presented in the following form:

$$D_a = A_\gamma \times F(\theta, t; \eta_{B,A}; \eta_{C,A}), \tag{4.6}$$

where F is a ratio of the right parts of Eqs. (4.5) and (4.3), θ the duration of exposure and t time after exposure; $\eta_{BA} = q_B/q_A$ and $\eta_{CA} = q_C/q_A$;

The direct correlation between the absorbed dose from alpha emitters ^{218}Po and ^{214}Po and beta- and gamma-emitters ^{214}Pb and ^{214}Bi in the lungs was first introduced in Ruzer (1958, 1960, 1968).

As a first step, it is important to know to what extent function F depends on the shift of equilibrium between ^{218}Po,^{214}Pb, and ^{214}Bi. The results of the calculations are presented in Table 4.1.

Table 4.1 Relationship between the function $F(\theta, \eta_{ba}, \eta_{ca})$ and the shift of equilibrium of radon decay products for various times of inhalation θ

η_{ba}, η_{ba}	$F(\theta, \eta_{ba}, \eta_{ba})$ $\theta = 3\eta$	$\times 10^4$ erg·min $\theta = 6\eta$
$\eta_{ba} = \eta_{ba} = 1$	23.8	47.8
$\eta_{ba} = \eta_{ba} = 0$	40.8	81.4
$\eta_{ba} = \eta_{ba} = 0.8$	24.2	48.2
$\eta_{ba} = \eta_{ba} = 0.6$	24.5	49
$\eta_{ba} = \eta_{ba} = 0.5$	24.9	49.8
$\eta_{ba} = \eta_{ba} = 0.4$	25.3	50.7
$\eta_{ba} = \eta_{ba} = 0.2$	27.2	54.5
$\eta_{ba} = \eta_{ba} = 0.1$	30	60
$\eta_{ba} = \eta_{ba} = 0.01$	38.2	75.8
$\eta_{ba} = 0.8; \eta_{ba} = 0.4$	24.5	48.8
$\eta_{ba} = 0.6; \eta_{ba} = 0.2$	25.3	50.5
$\eta_{ba} = 0.2; \eta_{ba} = 0.1$	28.2	56.3
$\eta_{ba} = 0.1; \eta_{ba} = 0.01$	32.2	64.4

Source: Copyright (2012). From *Aerosols Handbook: Measurement, Dosimetry, and Health Effects*, Second Edition, edited by Lev S. Ruzer and Naomi H. Harley. Reproduced by permission of Taylor and Francis Group, LLC, a division of Informa plc.

The results in Table 4.1 suggested that by measuring directly the gamma activity in the lungs, we could avoid the radon decay products concentration measurements. In this case, the maximum deviation from the mean value will be not more than 15%.

The final expression for the integral absorbed dose of alpha radiation for exposure time more than 3 h can be written as follows:

$$D_{\mathrm{a}} = 2.1 \times 10^{8} A_{\gamma} \times \theta \mathrm{erg}, \quad (4.7)$$

where θ is the duration of inhalation in hours and A_{γ} the activity of gamma-emitters in Ci.

For the maximum permissible concentration of 30 pCi/L (1100 Bq/m^3) [or in terms of (PAEC) 3.8 × 10^4 Mev/L], a breathing rate of 20 L/min and a standard lung deposition coefficient of 0.25 for a duration of 3 h or more the activity in the lungs will be about 0.02 μCi (740 Bq). This activity can be measured by external counting with good statistical accuracy. To prove this, model measurements were taken.

Results of measurement of the filtration ability of lungs are presented in Table 4.2.

4.3 Assessment of the Uncertainties in the Evaluation of the Dose

According to Ruzer (1970), the propagated errors in the calculation of the absorbed dose (exposure), based on measured air concentrations of decay products, is estimated to be at approximately 5–10 fold in comparison with the actual value of internal irradiation. Such large errors demand a special statistical treatment in the assessment of the dose. The assessment of the uncertainties in dose measurement was derived in Lekhtmakher et al. (1975).

Strictly speaking, a Gaussian function cannot serve to describe physical quantities whose domain is limited on the left. The contradiction is insignificant, however, when distribution dispersion remains low, as it also takes place in classical error theory. In the instance examined here, the conditions of low dispersion are violated.

Table 4.2 Measured air concentration of ^{214}Pb and ^{214}Bi gamma ray activity in miners' lungs and calculated filtration ability of lungs (FAL) for different groups of miners in a metal mine in Tadjikistan

Job category	Number of air samples	Concentration of ^{214}Pb + Bi (kBq.m^{-3}			No. of lung measurements	Activity in lungs (kBq)[a]			FAL = vk (m^3.min^{-1})			$FAL_{means}/FAL^{b}_{std}$	
		Average	Std error	Median		Average	Std error	Median	Average	Std error	Median	Average	Median
Drilling	92	5.92	0.55	3.7	219	2.66	0.22	2.59	0.0079	0.0014	0.0090	1.6	1.8
Auxiliary	76	6.88	0.81	5.2	104	2.63	0.30	1.92	0.0067	0.0015	0.0062	1.3	1.25
Inspection Personnel	129	11.1	1.11	7.4	68	3.26	0.33	2.11	0.0052	0.0011	0.0055	1.4	1.1
Average		8.9	0.9	5.2		2.85	0.26	2.22	0.0066	0.0011	0.0069	1.4	1.4

Source: Copyright (2012). From *Aerosols Handbook: Measurement, Dosimetry, and Health Effects*, Second Edition, edited by Lev S. Ruzer and Naomi H. Harley. Reproduced by permission of Taylor and Francis Group, LLC, a division of Informa plc.

[a]Actual gamma activities at the time of measurement. In calculating FAL, a correction was made on A_γ to account for decay between the end of the shift and the time of measurement, in all cases less than 1 h.

[b]FAL_{means} is the value based on the measured data, FAL_{std} is the calculated value based on the assumed standard breathing rate of 0.020 m^3·min^{-1} and standard fractional lung deposition of 0.25.

The expression for the absorbed dose D in the lungs over exposure time q can be presented by Eq. (4.5).

When we estimate the total error, it is necessary to take into account all partial errors such as the following:

1. correlation between the concentration in the respiratory zone and the site where sample was taken
2. variation in the concentration of radon progeny in the respiratory zone (up to 200%)
3. variation in the volumetric breathing rate and the lung deposition fraction during the work shift (up to 300%)

All these uncertainties will be even greater in calculation of the dose to the different part of the lungs, i.e., trachea, bronchi, etc., as other factors are involved.

Therefore in this case, when the error of the estimated activity in the lungs is so large, it is natural to suggest that the quantities found for the q, v and k can be, with equal probability, several times larger or smaller than the true values. A logarithmic normal distribution in this case is warranted. The magnitude of the activity will be log normally distributed according to a logarithmic normal law:

$$f(A)dA = 1/(2p)^{1/2} S_{\mathrm{g,A}} \times 1/A \times e^{-\mathrm{lg}2\times} A/A_{\mathrm{g}}/2S^2_{\mathrm{g,A}\times} dA, \quad (4.8)$$

where

$$A_{\mathrm{g}} = q_{\mathrm{g}} \times v_{\mathrm{g}} \times k_{\mathrm{g}} \times X(q) \text{ and } (S_{\mathrm{g,A}})^2 = (S_{\mathrm{g,q}})^2 + (S_{\mathrm{g,v}})^2 + (S_{\mathrm{g,k}})^2.$$

Supposing $S_{\mathrm{g,q}} = \ln 2$; $S_{\mathrm{g,v}} = \ln 3$; $S_{\mathrm{g,k}} = \ln 3$, we obtain

$$S_{\mathrm{g,A}} = 1.7.$$

This signifies that with a probability of 95% and 68%, respectively, the true value of A_{g} is between limits of $0.03A < A_{\gamma} < 30A$, and $0.18A < A_{\gamma} < 5.5A$, where A is the calculated value of the activity. The same magnitude of uncertainty will naturally be in the absorbed dose assessment. The results of this calculation suggested that the uncertainties in the dose assessment of miners are very high.

4.4 Correction for the Shift of Equilibrium of Radon Progeny in the Air and in the Lungs

The laboratory measurement of radon decay product gamma activity in simulated lungs was conducted using a calibrated sample of ^{226}Ra. The ^{226}Ra gamma spectrum is identical to the entire gamma-spectrum of radon progeny. However, there is a difference in the measurement performed on miners. In the ^{226}Ra calibration source, all radon decay products are in equilibrium, i.e., their activities are equal. The shift in equilibrium in the lungs will depend on the shift in equilibrium in the air and this will change with time in the lungs. This is especially important because the gamma-spectra of RaB and RaC are different, which will result in the change of gamma-detection efficiency with the change of equilibrium both in the air and in the lungs.

Let us denote the following:

e_0: Detection efficiency of RaB and RaC in equilibrium in the lungs or in the standard source of ^{226}Ra

e_b: Detection efficiency of RaB

$e_{c:}$ Detection efficiency of RaC

e: Detection efficiency in the case of the shift of equilibrium between RaB and RaC

$k_2(\theta,t) = e_0/e$: Correction factor on inequality of detection

Then,

$$e_0 = (N_{b,0} + N_{c,0})/2A_0, \quad (4.9)$$

where $N_{b,0}$ and $N_{c,0}$ are the count rates of RaB and RaC, respectively, from equilibrium RaB and RaC in the lungs or in the standard source of ^{226}Ra in the phantom, and A_0 the activity in the equilibrium source.

$$e = [N_b(\theta, t) + N_c(\theta, t)]/[A_b(\theta, t) + A_c(\theta, t)], \quad (4.10)$$

where N_b, N_c and A_b, A_c are the count rates and activities of RaB and RaC, respectively, in the lungs at time t after exposure time θ.

Then,

$$k_2 = e_0/e = (N_{b,0} + N_{c,0})/2A_0/(N_b + N_c)/(A_b + A_c);$$

$$N_{b,0} = e_b A_0;\ N_{c,0} = e_c A_c;$$

$$N_b = e_b A_b; N_c = e_c A_c;$$

$$k_2 = (e_b A_0 + e_c A_0)(A_c + A_b)/2A_0 \times (e_b A_b + e_c A_c). \quad (4.11)$$

And finally,

$$k_2(q, t) = (1 + e_c/e_b)(1 + A_c/A_b)/2[1 + (e_c/e_b)(A_c/A_b)]. \quad (4.12)$$

When the shift of equilibrium between RaA, RaB, and RAC in the air changes from 1:1:1 to 1:0.03: 0.01, the ratio of $A_c(t)/A_b(t)$ in the lungs changes from 0.31 to 2.93. However, due to the mode of the function k_2 (the ratios e_c/e_b and A_c/A_b are in both numerator and denominator), the difference in k_2 is not significant. For example, for a NaI(Tl)crystal 80 × 40 mm, the change in k_2 is not more than 20% (Ruzer and Urusov, 1969).

In calculating the detection efficiency for RaB and RaC, we have to take into account the number of gamma quanta per decay for RaB (0.823) and for RaC (1.397) with their average energies of 0.316 and 0.717 Mev, respectively.

Relative efficiency e_c/e_b was calculated for the 80 × 40 mm NaI(Tl) crystal and the model of the lungs (Ruzer and Urusov, 1969) according to the following formula:

$$e_c/e_b = \Sigma h_i \times k_{l,i} \times k_{b,i} \times k_{c,i}/\Sigma h_j \times k_{l,j} \times k_{b,j} \times k_{c,j}, \quad (4.13)$$

where h is the yield of the corresponding gamma-line, k_l, k_b the absorption coefficients of the lungs and the body, respectively, and k_c the detection efficiency of the crystal. The indexes i and j belong to RaC and RaB, respectively.

Simplifying the expression for the average absorbed dose, assuming that the mass m of the lung is 1000 g,

$$D/m = 8.05 \times 10^{-7} k_1 \times k_2 \times k_3 N_{0,\gamma} \times \theta \text{ mrad}, \quad (4.14)$$

where θ is the duration of the inhalation, $N_{0,\gamma}$ the count rate above the "background" (the "background" is the count rate measured for the person before entering working place), k_1 the correction coefficient for decay of radon progeny in lungs after the end of

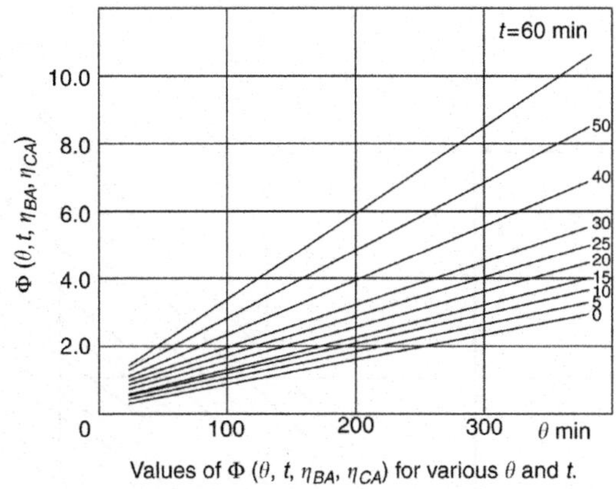

Figure 4.1 Values of Φ $(\theta, t, \eta_{ba}, \eta_{ca})$ for various θ and t. Copyright (2012). From *Aerosols Handbook: Measurement, Dosimetry, and Health Effects*, Second Edition, edited by Lev S. Ruzer and Naomi H. Harley. Reproduced by permission of Taylor and Francis Group, LLC, a division of Informa plc.

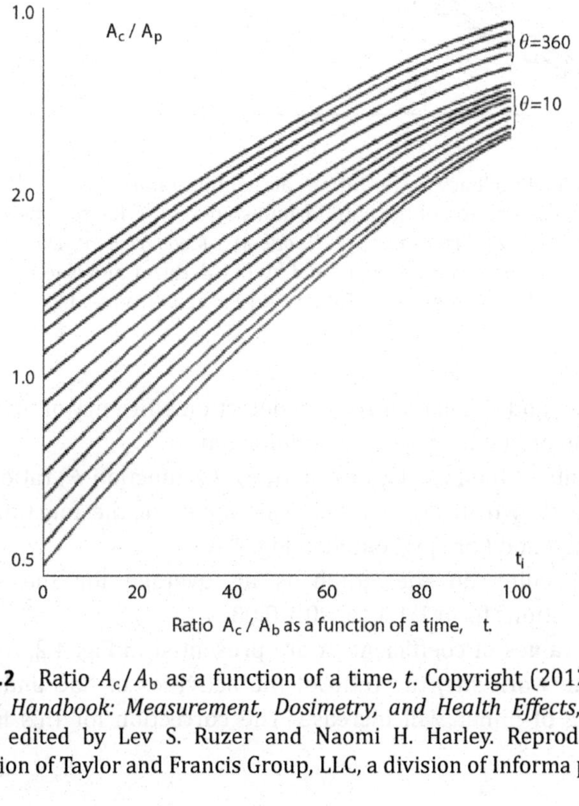

Figure 4.2 Ratio A_c/A_b as a function of a time, t. Copyright (2012). From *Aerosols Handbook: Measurement, Dosimetry, and Health Effects*, Second Edition, edited by Lev S. Ruzer and Naomi H. Harley. Reproduced by permission of Taylor and Francis Group, LLC, a division of Informa plc.

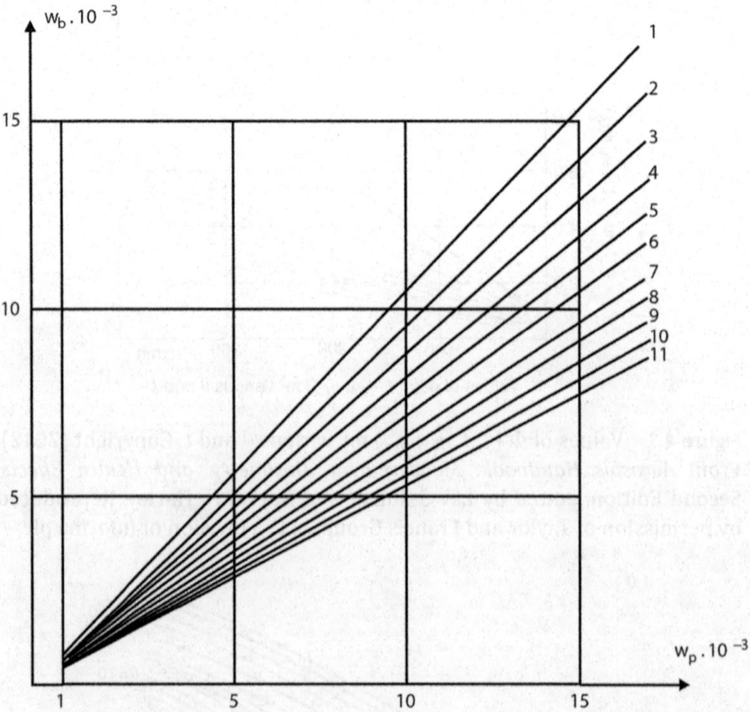

Figure 4.3 Efficiency registration of gamma-radiation of ^{214}Pb e_b vs. efficiency registration of the equilibrium source of ^{226}Ra for different e_c/e_b. Copyright (2012). From *Aerosols Handbook: Measurement, Dosimetry, and Health Effects*, Second Edition, edited by Lev S. Ruzer and Naomi H. Harley. Reproduced by permission of Taylor and Francis Group, LLC, a division of Informa plc.

exposure, and k_3 the reciprocal of detection efficiency of the gamma radiation of radon progeny in equilibrium.

Results of the calculations of k_1, k_2, k_3, function F, ratio A_c/A_b, etc., are shown in Fig. 4.1–4.5. The values of the function F for different θ and t are presented in Fig. 4.1.

Each point on the graph is an average for the shift of concentrations from 1:1:1 to 1:0.1:0.03:

The values of coefficients k are presented in Fig. 4.2. After exit from the work site, the ratio of the activities of RaC and RaB in the lung of miner will increase. The correction for this factor is

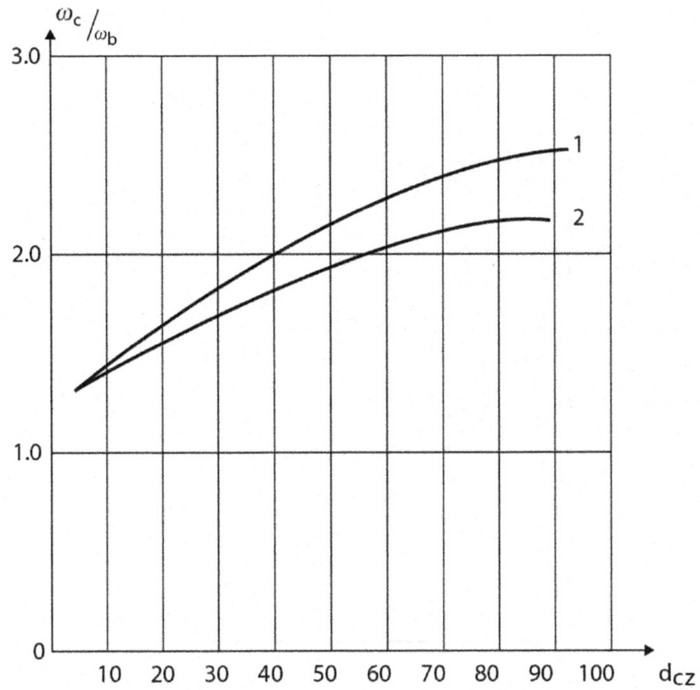

Figure 4.4 Ratio e_c/e_b as a function of crystal thickness (mm): (1) source of ^{226}Ra; (2) registration from the chest. Copyright (2012). From *Aerosols Handbook: Measurement, Dosimetry, and Health Effects*, Second Edition, edited by Lev S. Ruzer and Naomi H. Harley. Reproduced by permission of Taylor and Francis Group, LLC, a division of Informa plc.

substantial, when direct measurement is not provided immediately after exit from the working site. The ratio of the activities of RaC (^{214}Bi) and ^{214}Pb (RaB) at time after exposure is presented in Fig. 4.3.

The efficiency of registration of the gamma ray from ^{214}Pb depends on the size of the crystal and the geometrical (position) factor. The dependency of the efficiency, e_b, of the gamma radiation of ^{214}Pb from the ^{226}Ra for different equilibrium ratios, e_c/e_b, are shown in Fig. 4.4.

The ratio e_c/e_b as a function of the crystal thickness (mm) (1) ^{226}Ra source and (2) registration from the chest) is presented in Fig. 4.4.

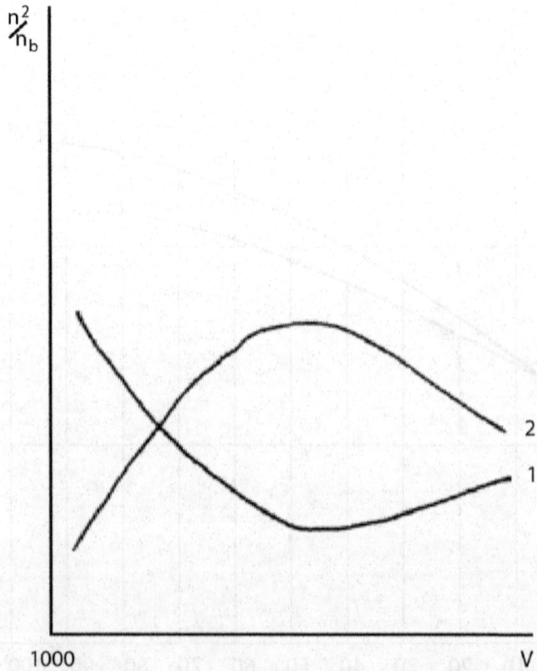

Figure 4.5 Statistical error (1) and the quality factor (2) vs. voltage on the photomultiplier (Ruzer, 2001). Copyright (2012). From *Aerosols Handbook: Measurement, Dosimetry, and Health Effects*, Second Edition, edited by Lev S. Ruzer and Naomi H. Harley. Reproduced by permission of Taylor and Francis Group, LLC, a division of Informa plc.

It should be pointed out that measurement of the gamma-activity in the lungs of miners was provided in the environment with relatively high gamma-background, especially when measurements took place near the working sites. In such cases, the parameter "quality of measurement" $q = n^2/n_b$ (where n is the count rate above the background and n_b the background count rate) was chosen to achieve the best measurements conditions. The results of this study are shown in Figs. 4.5 and 4.6.

Figure 4.5 shows the statistical error (1) and the "quality factor" (2) vs. the voltage on the photomultiplier (FEA). Figure 4.6 shows the statistical error (1) and the "quality factor" (2) vs. amplification coefficient.

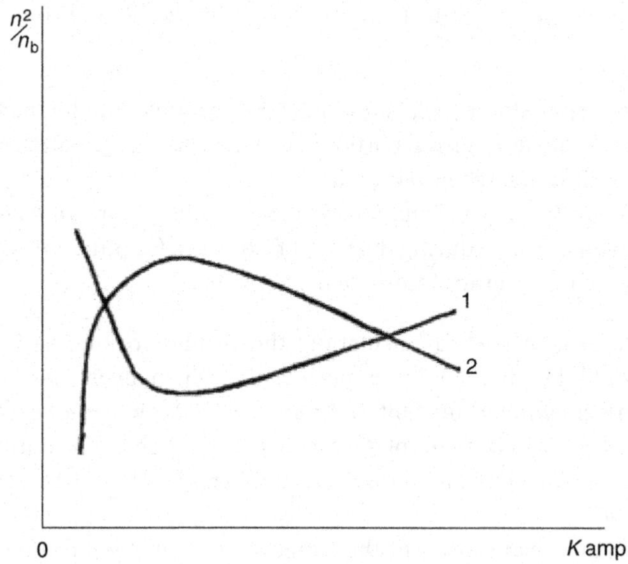

Figure 4.6 Statistical error (1) and the quality factor (2) vs. amplification coefficient. Copyright (2012). From *Aerosols Handbook: Measurement, Dosimetry, and Health Effects*, Second Edition, edited by Lev S. Ruzer and Naomi H. Harley. Reproduced by permission of Taylor and Francis Group, LLC, a division of Informa plc.

4.5 Accounting for Parametric Variations: Variations of Concentrations, Breathing Rate and Deposition Coefficients in Real Working Conditions

All dosimetric parameters under actual working conditions are not uniform. This is important both in the case of the estimated or indirect calculation of the dose (lung activity) and in the case of direct measurement.

Let us denote Q (the activity in the lung) as a combination of all parameters (air concentration, breathing rate, lung deposition, respirator efficiency):

$$Q = qvk(1 - f), \tag{4.15}$$

where f is the coefficient of effectiveness of a respirator and Q the rate of the intake.

To take into account the variation of intake, two options were used:

(a) Experimental, by placing a portable gamma-counter near the work site and for the parts of the shift with special attention to the situation when Q is high.
(b) Theoretical, by calculation of corresponding corrections on the inequality of Q during the time of exposure for different types of working itinerary (scenario of exposure).

To perform such a calculation, the whole working shift time, θ, should be divided by n periods in which every dosimetric parameters will be constant. Different typical scenarios of exposure (work itinerary) in terms of the rate of intake, Q, changing during the shift were calculated in Gerasimov and Ruzer (1973) and presented in Fig. 4.7.

Variant 1 can represent the situation on Monday morning since the ventilation was usually turned off over the weekend. This resulted in increasing q and, consequently, Q.

Variants 7 and 8 present situations during the work shift:

(a) ventilation was turned off (on) which resulted in increasing (decreasing) q,
(b) change in physico-chemical properties of aerosols that result in an increase (decrease) of the coefficient k,
(c) change in the work load resulting in changed breathing rate and deposition coefficient,
(d) miners' use of respirators resulting in a change of the factor $1-f$.

For the introduction of a correction factor for Q, we have to get additional information on each concrete working situation (variation of Q during the shift). The degree of the error in determining the correction factor depends on the proximity of the chosen variant of the function Q to the variant under actual conditions.

According to the calculations (Urusov 1972), even if the magnitude of Q_{max}/Q_{min} is close to 30, the total error in the measurement of activity in the lungs of miners by the direct method will not exceed 40%, which is acceptable for the purposes of individual dosimetry.

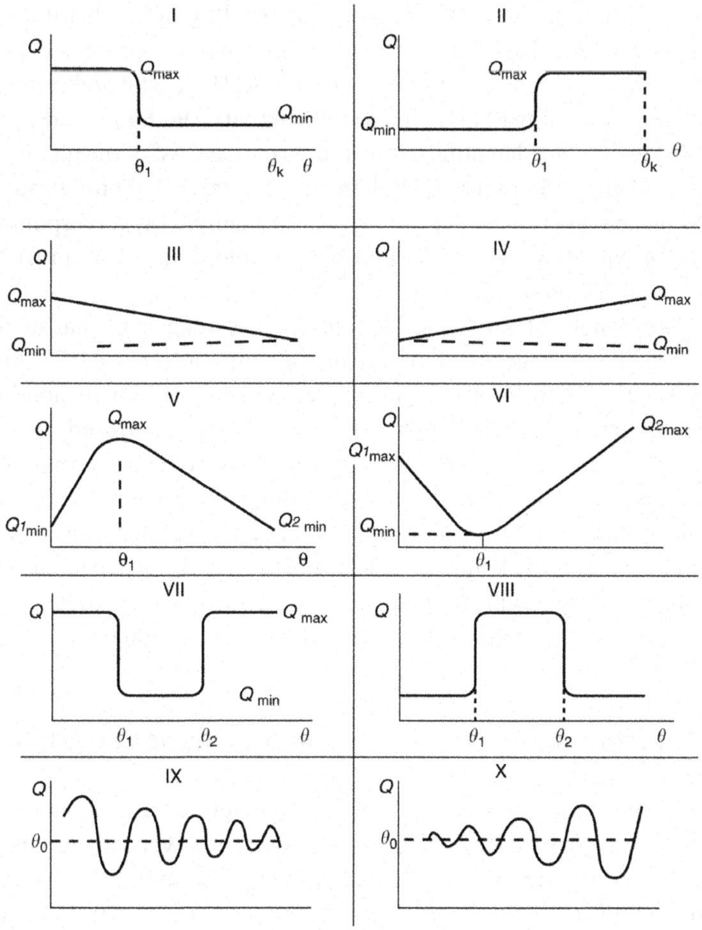

Figure 4.7 Type of function (Q). Copyright (2012). From *Aerosols Handbook: Measurement, Dosimetry, and Health Effects*, Second Edition, edited by Lev S. Ruzer and Naomi H. Harley. Reproduced by permission of Taylor and Francis Group, LLC, a division of Informa plc.

4.6 Model Measurement

Experiments to determine the detection limit of the gamma-activity measurement of radon progeny in the lungs of miners were provided using a Human Body Spectrometer at the Biophysics Institute in Moscow. It consisted of a measurement chamber protected by a 20 cm layer of iron. The detector was a NaI(Tl) crystal and samples of ^{226}Ra containing $RaCl_2$ solution with activity 590 Bq (a) and 175.4 Bq (b) were placed in different positions in the chest of the phantom, and a 80 mm × 50 mm NaI(Tl) detection crystal and photomultiplier was placed on the back. The activity of the sample (a) corresponded to approximately 0.75 of Annual Permissible Concentration (APC) and (b) 0.25 APC in air.

The results of these model experiments suggested that at the level of concentration of radon progeny in the air of 0.75 APC, 4.3×10^4 MeV/L (or correspondingly 30 pCi/L), the corresponding gamma-activity in the lungs of miners can be measured by one detector within 3 min with an accuracy of 8%, if the measurement of the background was 10 min. Even if we take into account that in real underground conditions measurements take place 30–40 min after completing the work during which time the activity will decrease by a factor of two, it will still be possible to measure the activity in the lungs with an accuracy of 15% for a measurement of 5 min.

4.7 Phantom Measurements and Geometric Corrections

For calibration purposes in laboratory conditions, a phantom of the human torso was used. The measurements were made with a NaI(Tl) crystal with a window diameter of 77 mm, a lead shield and cylindrical sample of ^{226}Ra activity of 3.9×10^{-5} Ci size 160 × 16 mm placed in different positions in the phantom.

Results of phantom measurements, including positions of the sample and the detector, are shown in Table 4.3. Measurements were provided by scintillation detector of NaI(Tl) with lead shield (diameter of the window 77 mm).

For the field measurements, a more primitive phantom was used, i.e., a long-sized vessel filled with water and size close to the size of lungs, in which the sources of ^{226}Ra were places in different positions.

The systematic errors associated with the contamination of the body and work clothes in real working conditions for example,

Table 4.3 Phantom measurements

i/*j*	1	2	3
1	3500	450	50
2	1600	600	130
3	2200	1050	130
4	1550	1350	110
5	620	800	460
6	750	1400	470
7	600	1900	400
8	100	650	3650

Source: Copyright (2012). From *Aerosols Handbook: Measurement, Dosimetry, and Health Effects*, Second Edition, edited by Lev S. Ruzer and Naomi H. Harley. Reproduced by permission of Taylor and Francis Group, LLC, a division of Informa plc.
Note: i, detector position; j, source of ^{226}Ra position.

the influence of radon accumulated in the adipose tissue of the abdominal cavity was eliminated by the introduction of corresponding corrections. It has been shown that the contribution of gamma radiation from the abdomen to the total count rate 30 min after leaving the working place does not exceed 5%.

The errors associated with the contamination of the clothes and the body of miners dropped to 15% and 1% of the measured value, respectively, after work clothes had been taken off and a shower was taken. The variability of the background in underground measurements with the same person was no more than 3%.

The dependence of the gamma-background on the body thickness is shown in Fig. 4.8.

The decay of radon progeny in the lungs of miners is presented in Fig. 4.9. The figure shows that the activity in the lung of miners decreased according to the law of radioactive decay of radon progeny, i.e., no substantial clearance was found during the 3 h period.

The dependence of the count rate from the distance between the detector and the chest is shown in Fig. 4.10, where a is the efficiency of registration, b is the statistical error, 1 refers to one detector with a single window, 2 refers to one detector with a double window, and 3 refers to two detectors with a double window.

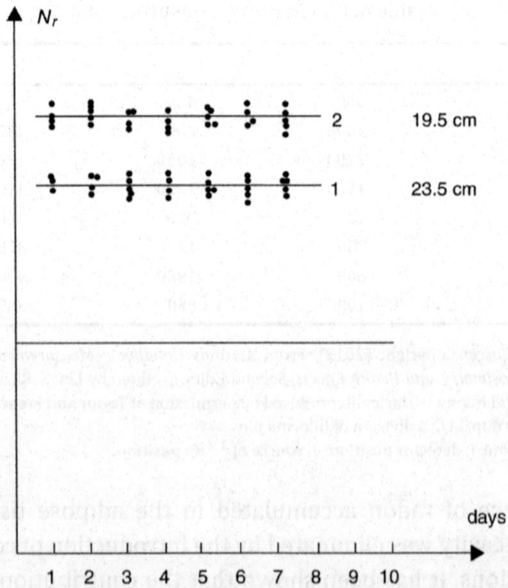

Figure 4.8 Dependence of gamma-background on body thickness. Copyright (2012). From *Aerosols Handbook: Measurement, Dosimetry, and Health Effects*, Second Edition, edited by Lev S. Ruzer and Naomi H. Harley. Reproduced by permission of Taylor and Francis Group, LLC, a division of Informa plc.

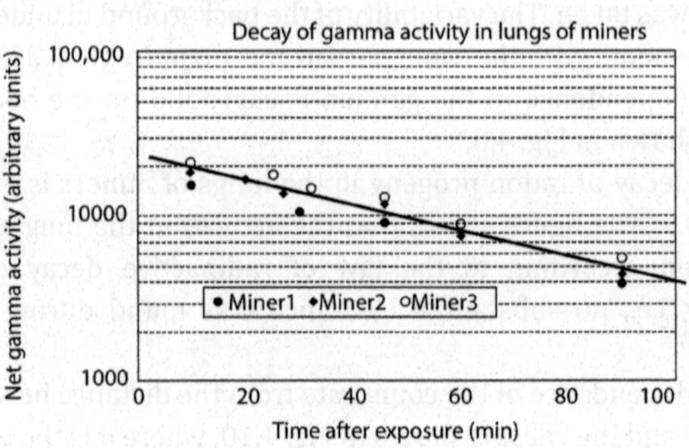

Figure 4.9 Decay of gamma activity in the lungs of miners. Copyright (2012). From *Aerosols Handbook: Measurement, Dosimetry, and Health Effects*, Second Edition, edited by Lev S. Ruzer and Naomi H. Harley. Reproduced by permission of Taylor and Francis Group, LLC, a division of Informa plc.

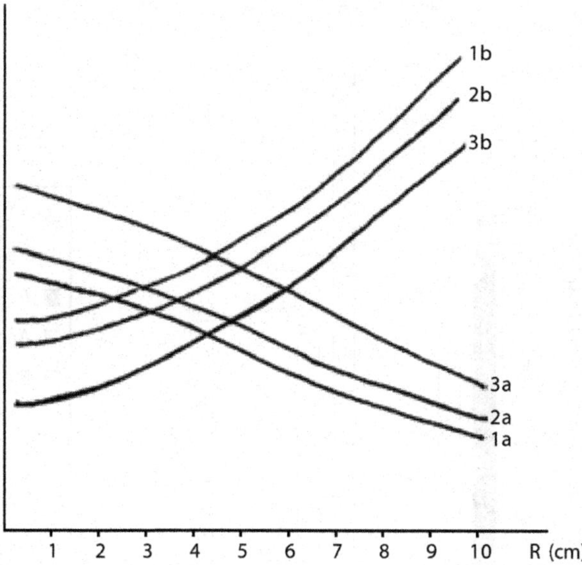

Figure 4.10 Dependence of the efficiency (a) and statistical error (b) from the distance of the body from the detector. Copyright (2012). From *Aerosols Handbook: Measurement, Dosimetry, and Health Effects*, Second Edition, edited by Lev S. Ruzer and Naomi H. Harley. Reproduced by permission of Taylor and Francis Group, LLC, a division of Informa plc.

Dependency of the count rate from the horizontal (x) and vertical (z) shift of the body for one (I) and two (II) detectors is shown in Fig. 4.11.

4.8 Assessment of the Errors of the Direct Method

As it is obvious from Eq. (4.15) that the errors associated with direct measurement of activity of radon progeny in the lungs depends on many factors; each of them should be studied carefully:

(1) error associated with the measurement of activity in the lungs, including geometrical factors, quality of measurement factor, etc. (δ_1)
(2) error associated with the contamination of the body and clothes of miners (δ_2)

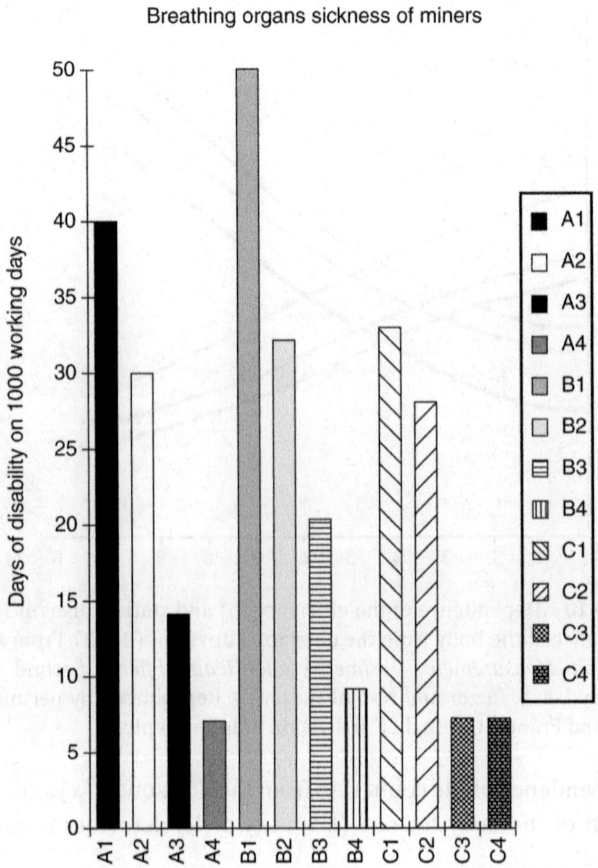

Figure 4.11 Sickness of different groups of miners in terms of the days of disability for two periods of observation with the higher and lower concentration: 1—high exposure (radon decay product concentration), general number of days of sickness 2—low exposure (radon decay product concentration), general number of days of sickness 3—high exposure, days in a hospital; A—for all miners, B—for drillers, C—for others. Copyright (2012). From *Aerosols Handbook: Measurement, Dosimetry, and Health Effects*, Second Edition, edited by Lev S. Ruzer and Naomi H. Harley. Reproduced by permission of Taylor and Francis Group, LLC, a division of Informa plc.

(3) errors associated with calculation of the coefficients k_2 and k_3, respectively (δ_3, δ_4)
(4) errors associated with variation of Q during the time of exposure (δ_5)
(5) errors associated with the averagination of the function F (δ_6)
(6) errors associated with the uncertainty of the times of exposure and the time t (δ_7) (δ_8).

Calculations show that for the measurement using a crystal size of 80 $\times$ 40 mm with the average radon progeny concentration equal to 3.9 $\times$ 10^4 Mev/L will not exceed 26%.

Under mining conditions, it is necessary to take into account the contamination of the body and clothing of miners by radon decay products; otherwise the systematic error of measurement activity in the lung can be very high. The study showed that in radon decay products measurements in lungs of miners with the clothes taken off, δ_2, decreases to 16%, and after shower was taken, δ_2, decreases to 1%. The error in determination of k_2 - δ_3 does not exceed 2%.

The error δ_4, which is a characteristic of the degree of the difference between real situation and measurement in lungs, includes in itself the error in the measurement of the activity in the standard source of Ra-226, $\delta_{4,1}$; error related to difference between the size of the real chest and the average that was taken into account in calculation $\delta_{4,2}$; and errors $\delta_{4,3}$ and $\delta_{4,4}$ associated with position of the body to the detector and in non-uniformity of distribution of activity in the lungs. The error $\delta_{4,1}$ was not more than 3%. The assessment of $\delta_{4,2}$ was $\delta_{4,3}$ in the chest size measurements of miners and also in the study of the correlation between the vertical and horizontal changes of position of the body and the count rate. The results showed that $\delta_{4,2}$ = 5% and $\delta_{4,3}$ = 10%. The assessment of $\delta_{4,4}$ was based on the fact (Urusov, 1972) that non-uniformity in the activity distribution in the lungs does not exceed 30%. The calculation of this error was determined theoretically by using the lung model, represented by two cylinders in a case when the activity in one of one 1/4 of the cylinder was change by 30%. In this case, the error $\delta_{4,4}$ was 5%. Therefore δ_4 was 12%.

Evaluation of δ_5 presents special difficulties, for it requires additional information associated with the work itinerary (scenario of exposure), i.e., type of the function Q.

For this assessment, the measurements of radon decay product concentrations were made at 208 working sites. In 98% of the cases, q_{max}/q_{min} does not exceed 5 with the maximum of 9.

Taking into account the difference in the breathing rate, the ratio of Q_{max}/Q_{min} was 15. If we suppose that the changes in Q within the shift takes place not more than 10 times within the shift, δ_5 will be no more than 30% for $Q_{max}/Q_{min} = 15$.

The error δ_6 was no more than 3% with known θ and t. An error associated with known θ – δ_7 in the real working situation was no more than 4%. The uncertainty in the time (t) if the instruction of workers was made with the periodic control of the time of leaving the working site should be not more than 5 min in terms of time and consequently 9% as an error. Thus, the resulting error in the measurement of radon decay products activity in the lungs of miners in real mining environment will be

$$\delta = \sqrt{(\delta_1)^2 + (\delta_2)^2 + (\delta_3)^2 + (\delta_4)^2 + (\delta_5)^2 + (\delta_6)^2 + (\delta_7)^2 + (\delta_8)^2}. \tag{4.16}$$

For the average PAEC of 1.3×10^5 Mev/L (1 working level), δ will be near 38% and for 3.9×10^4 Mev/L correspondingly 50%. These results were confirmed by the measurement in real underground conditions. Similar calculations were provided for thoron decay products and for the mixture of radon and thoron.

According to Urusov (1972), the level of thoron decay products in non-uranium mines in Tadjikistan was on average 10 times lower than for radon progeny. All coefficients and formulas in the case of thoron and radon decay products mixture will be similar to what it was in the case of radon progeny itself.

In the case of thoron + radon decay products, the measurement of the activity can be provided by sequential gamma ray activity due to difference in the half-time decay of each family. Ten hours after miners' exit from the working site, the activity of radon decay products will be 0.1% from that in the moment of the end of the work, while the thoron decay products are at the original activity.

The background measurement should be provided for each miner using the maximum interval between two shifts, for example, on Monday, when the activity of thoron daughters will be 1% of that in the moment of leaving working place on Friday.

4.9 Portable Instrument for Direct Measurement of the Activity of Radon Decay Products in the Lungs of Miners

Some variants of portable instruments were developed for measuring miners both near the working sites and in the sanitary building, where miners took showers and changed their working clothes. Instruments with one and two detectors (for the front and back of the chest) were developed. For field measurement, NaI(Tl) crystals were used with standard lead blocks as a shield. The main demand on the instrument was to measure the concentration of radon progeny at a concentration of 1.3×10^5 Mev/L (1 WL) and taking into account the general tendency of decreasing the maximum permissible concentration even on the level of 3.9×10^4 Mev/L (0.3 WL). The radiometric quality of the instrumentation can be improved by increasing counting efficiency by using a crystal of larger size, higher density CsI(Tl), or semiconductor detectors, or by decreasing the background. A study of the correlation between background and shield thickness has shown that after increasing the thickness above 5 cm, no decrease of the background took place. Therefore, 5 cm thickness of the lead shield was chosen as optimal (Urusov, 1972).

The measurement of activity in the lungs can be provided by means of general gamma activity measurement or spectrometry. The calculation shows that the quality factor of the first group of measurement is higher.

A portable instrument for direct measurement was used that allowed transport very close to the working site and performed measurements within 1–2 min, without interruption of work.

More than 500 measurements of the activity (dose) in the lungs of miners were provided in uranium and non-uranium mines of former Middle Asia Republics of the USSR over an 11-year period.

Table 4.4 Measurements of the activity (dose) in the lungs of miners

Names	1	2	3 N_0	4 N	5	6
ä-v	420	20	574	671	17,0	55
V-n	420	25	574	667	17,0	57
S-v	420	25	574	638	16,0	39
ä-v	420	25	574	664	16,0	55
O-v"	420	25	574	609	3,0	21
ï-v"	420	25	574	614	3,0	24
ë-Í	420	30	574	614	4,0	26
Ñ-Ó"	420	30	574	608	4,0	22
ë-n"	420	30	574	604	13,0	20
F-v	420	30	574	613	13,0	26
ë-n	420	40	574	562	14,0	0
L-i"	420	30	574	550	14,0	0
ë- i"	420	30	574	609	13,0	23
I-Ó"	420	30	574	615	4,0	26
V-n	420	25	574	586	3,0	0
K-n"	420	20	574	680	17,0	60
S-j	420	20	574	681	17,0	61
S-n	420	25	574	671	16,0	59

Source: Copyright (2012). From *Aerosols Handbook: Measurement, Dosimetry, and Health Effects*, Second Edition, edited by Lev S. Ruzer and Naomi H. Harley. Reproduced by permission of Taylor and Francis Group, LLC, a division of Informa plc.
Note: N_0, background count rate, i.e., before entering radon atmosphere; N, count rate after leaving working site; 1, time of exposure, min; 2, time of measurement, min; 3, 4, counts rates (multiplied by 16); 5, PAEC, MeV/l; 6, absorbed dose, mrad.

Some of the results are presented in Table 4.4. Measurements took place in June 1969 in Tadjikistan (former USSR).

The measurements reported here were carried out in a non-uranium mine in Tadjikistan with a special instrument containing two probes, with a similar counting of 1.8 or 3.6 diameter filtered samples with a ZnS scintillation probe.

The measurement of gamma activity deposited in the lung was performed using a low background gamma probe consisting of a collimated 80 × 40 mm NaI (Tl) crystal in 50 mm of lead shielding. The background counting rate was determined by measuring each miner before entering the work area. Miners pressed their chests to the window of the NaI (Tl) detector after removing their outer clothing and gamma count rate was measured. A similar measurement was taken after leaving the workplace, and deposited activity in the lung was calculated from the net count rate.

As presented above, the theory, model measurements, corrections, assessment of the errors, and results of measurements on miners suggested that even using portable instruments, it is possible to measure the activity of radon decay products in the lungs of miners at a level even lower than the APC.

By using such a technique, it was possible to introduce actual individual dosimetry for hundreds of thousands of underground workers in mines where the levels of radon were similar to that found in non-uranium mines in Tadjikistan.

Besides this, direct measurement presents an opportunity for the non-invasive measurement of the filtration ability of lungs (FAL)—value responsible for aerosol deposition in lungs. This value, which is a "bridge" between concentration in the air and deposited aerosol activity (or mass) in the lungs, plays an important part in the inhaled particles dosimetry for all kind of aerosols. The uncertainty in FAL measurement is much lower than in the determination of breathing volume rate and deposition coefficient separately.

As it is known, the biological effect of aerosols depends on the local dose, because sensitivity of the lung tissue to different substances, deposition, clearance, and transport of deposited aerosols inside the lung is not uniform. In this connection, the local FAL (LFAL) is an important parameter to correlate dose with the concentration for both radioactive and nonradioactive aerosols.

It should be also mentioned that radon decay products are good natural marker owing to their short-lived nature and relatively high permissible concentration in comparison with the most of artificial aerosols.

In mines, the primitive portable technique was used due to special underground conditions.

By studying the deposition of aerosols in lungs with radon progeny as a marker in laboratory conditions and by using spectrometric detectors, scanners, and three-dimensional techniques, it is possible to study experimentally, not by modeling, the deposition of aerosols in different parts of the lung for different particle size distribution.

References

Bateman H (1910) *Proc Cambridge Phil Soc* **15**, 423.

Gerasimov YS, Ruzer LS (1973) Methods of determining the amount of radioactive isotopes in human organism. Symposium Materials. Leningrad NII Radiation Hygiene, Leningrad, p. 58.

Lekhtmakher SO, Ruzer LS (1975) *Izmer Tekhn* **5**.

Ruzer LS (1958) *Atomnaya Energiya* February, 189–194.

Ruzer LS (1960) *Atomnaya Energiya* **8**(6), 557–559.

Ruzer LS (1968) *Radioactive Aerosols*, Moscow, 191 pp. (in Russian).

Ruzer LS (1970) Radioactive aerosols: Determination of the absorbed dose, doctoral dissertation, Moscow, USSR.

Ruzer LS, Nero AV, Harley NH (1995) *Radiat Prot Dosimetry* **58**, 261–265.

Ruzer LS, Urusov SA (1969) *Atomnaya Energiya* **26**, 301–303.

Urusov SA (1972) Method and measurement technique for determination of the intake of radon decay products in the lungs of underground workers, Candidate's Dissertation. Biophysics Institute of the USSR Minstry of Health, Moscow (in Russian).

Chapter 5

Assessment of the Nanoparticles' Surface Area by Measuring the Unattached Activity of Radon Progeny

The proposed method represents a synthesis of

1. derived direct analytical correlation between "unattached fraction" of radon progeny and surface area particle concentration in the range of 1–100 nm particle diameter, and
2. experimental data on correlation between the unattached fraction of radon progeny and particle surface area with diameter in the range of 44 nm to 2.1 μm.

A review of the literature on the environment health implications of the developing nanotechnology industry shows that the potential problem of exposure to nanoparticles has led to elevated concentrations of nanomaterials and has not been adequately assessed (Oberdörster et al., 2005). The health and safety of nanotechnology workers is of concern because these groups are likely to be exposed to elevated concentrations of nanomaterials. A gap exists between currently available particle measurement methods and those appropriate for nanoaerosol exposure measurement. Two

Nanoparticles in Humans: Experiments, Methods, and Strategies
Lev S. Ruzer

ISBN 978-981-4463-16-4 (Hardcover), 978-981-4463-17-1 (eBook)
www.panstanford.com

main types of instruments for measuring the airborne concentration of nanoparticle have been used: condensation particle counters (CPDs) and differential mobility analyzers (DMA).

Particle counting efficiencies of a condensation particle counter (TSI CPC 3762) under different operating parameters were presented by Banse et al. (2001). This study showed a substantial decrease in the detection efficiency for particles in the size range 6–10 nm. Concentration measurements of nanoparticles by differential mobility analyzers suffer low counting efficiency mainly due to the low probability with which nanoparticles are charged (NSF, 2003).

A number of studies on the exposure of nanoparticles have indicated that health effects associated with low-solubility inhaled nanometer aerosols may be more appropriately associated with particle surface area than with mass concentration (Donaldson et al., 1998; Oberdörster, 2005). Data on the correlation between particle number, surface area, and mass concentration and human health effects are needed for exposure investigations, but the means for measuring aerosol surface area are not readily available.

A new instrument, the Nanoparticle Surface Area Monitor (TSI 3550, Nanoparticle Surface Area Monitor, 2005) uses the previously developed TSI Model 3070 Electrical Aerosol Detector (EAD) for the assessment of deposited surface area (DSA) in the lung. Lung deposition estimates made by this instrument are based on correlations between the electrical signal and calculated DSA (Wilson et al., 2004). The manufacturer claims that this instrument is capable of detecting particles as small as 10 nm. Another method of assessing nanoparticle surface area is based on the simultaneous measurement of number and mass concentrations (Maynard, 2003).

The main existing methods used in the assessment of airborne nanoparticle in the range of 1–10 nm concentration are

- injection of saturated vapor into the measured volume with subsequent measurement of aerosols formed due to condensation of the vapor onto nanoparticles;
- application of electrical charge to the measured volume with subsequent quantification of nanoparticle deposition;
- light scattering of nanoparticles.

In this chapter, we discuss a different approach to the measurement of aerosol surface area concentration, based on the use of the radioactive inert gas radon and its decay products. This method relies on the deposition of the "unattached activity fraction of radon progeny" on aerosol particles.

5.1 The Unattached Activity of Radon Decay Products

One important property of radon decay products is that after alpha decay of radon, the newly formed atom of ^{218}Po becomes surrounded by a small number of molecules (around 10 to 12). Such molecular clusters, referred to as unattached progeny, with sizes in the range 1–4 nm and diffusion coefficients of approximately 0.06 cm^2 s^{-1}, can be potentially useful as a marker in the studies of properties of non-radioactive aerosols, especially nanoaerosols. Figure 5.1 depicts the basic processes of gaseous radon decay producing unattached progeny. These progeny may remain unattached, or may become associated with existing aerosols. It seems reasonable that there should be some correlation between unattached activity and aerosol concentration. It is likely that lower aerosol concentrations will lead to larger fractions of unattached

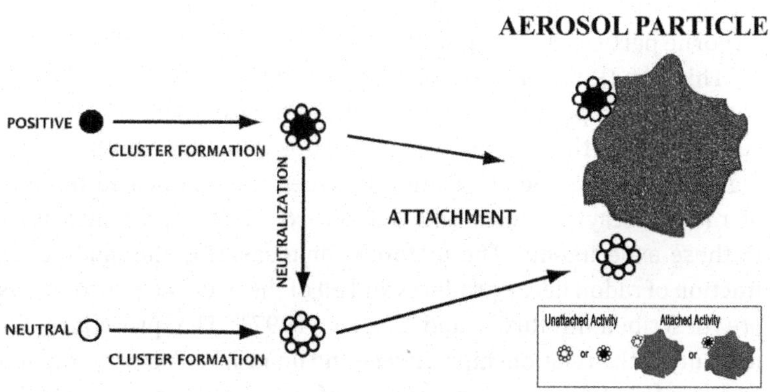

Figure 5.1 Basic processes of Rn decay behavior in air, defining "unattached" and "aerosol attached" activities. Clusters that do not attach to an aerosol particle are called "unattached fraction."

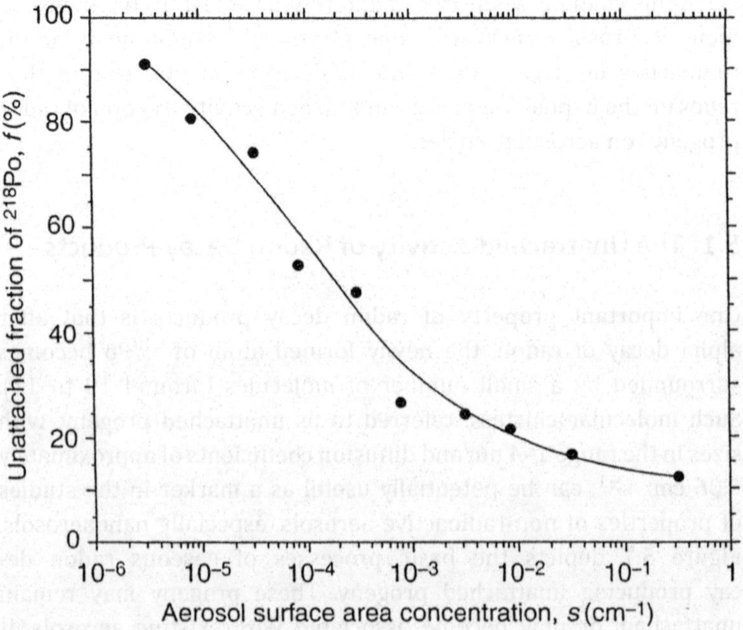

Figure 5.2 Correlation between nanoaerosols surface area and unattached fraction.

activity. If this relationship can be quantified, then the unattached activity fraction of radon progeny can be used as a measure of airborne particle concentration.

This idea (Ruzer, 1964) was illustrated by an experimental study with spherical polystyrene particles in the size range 0.3–2.1 μm, i.e., outside of the nanometer range (Dokukina and Ruzer, 1976). Figure 5.2 shows the correlation between the unattached fraction of radon decay products and the aerosol surface area measured in these experiments. The methods for measuring the unattached fraction of radon decay products and all of the necessary corrections are described in Ruzer and Sextro (1997). The procedure for measuring the relationship between the unattached activity fraction and particle concentration consists of passing the radon-exposed air through a device with two channels: one with only an open filter and the other with a diffusion battery or other sampler for unattached radon decay products (for example, the wire screen) preceding a particle filter. The calibration procedure includes the determination of five parameters. First, the deposition efficiency in the diffusion battery of the unattached, e_1, and attached, e_2, activities is determined. Then the detection efficiency in the diffusion battery of the unattached, e_3, and attached, e_4, activities is determined. Finally, the detection efficiency of the open filter, e, is determined.

The measurement of these parameters should be provided by means of an "unattached activity generator," a device capable of generating a regulated unattached activity fraction. Such generators were described in Dokukina and Ruzer (1976) and Butterweck et al. (2001). The formula for the unattached fraction of radon decay products, i.e., the ratio of the unattached activity to the total (unattached + attached) airborne activity of radon decay products f (Ruzer and Sextro, 1997) is

$$f = Ae/N_{of} = [eN_{db}(1 - e_2) - e_2e_4N_{bf}]/N_{of}[e_1e_3(1 - e_2) - e_2e_4(1 - e_1)], \quad (5.1)$$

where A is the activity of the unattached fraction and N_{of}, N_{db}, and N_{bf} are the number counts for the open filter, diffusion battery, and filter behind the diffusion battery, respectively.

Deposition processes for unattached radon decay products to aerosol particles have been studied both theoretically and experimentally (Lassen and Rau, 1960; Lassen and Weicksel, 1960). Their work showed that for particles smaller than 10 nm, the probability of deposition attachment is proportional to the square of the particle radius, and for particles larger than 1 μm, deposition is proportional to the particle radius. Those studies determined the general formula for the constant of deposition, λ_{at}, of the unattached activity to aerosol particles in equilibrium to be

$$\lambda_{at} = (1/\tau) = 4\pi r^2 N\beta/(1 + hr) = S\beta/(1 + rh), \quad (5.2)$$

where τ is the time for the concentration of unattached activity to decrease by a factor of $1/e$, r is the particle radius, N is the particle number concentration, $\beta = (v/4) \sim 4300$ cm s^{-1}, $h = v/4\pi D \sim 70000$ cm^{-1} and S is the particle surface area concentration. Here, v is the root-mean-square velocity of radon decay product molecules under standard conditions and D is the Brownian diffusion coefficient of the unattached particles.

Croft and Perry (1962) described the formation of the unattached activity from radon and its deposition onto aerosol particles and surfaces. They developed the following expression for the unattached activity fraction f:

$$f = \lambda_A/(\lambda_A + \lambda_{at}), \tag{5.3}$$

where λ_A is the decay constant of ^{218}Po, the first daughter product of radon decay. Combining Eqs. (5.2) and (5.3) yields Eq. (5.4), an expression that directly correlates aerosol surface area, S, to the unattached activity fraction f:

$$S = (\lambda_A/\beta)[(1/f) - 1](1 + rh) \tag{5.4}$$

For particles in the size range 1–100 nm, the term $(1 + rh)$ is approximately equal to 1, and equation (5.4) can be simplified to

$$S = (\lambda_A/\beta)[(1/f) - 1]. \tag{5.5}$$

Results calculated for ^{218}Po by means of Eq. (5.5) that show the relationship of the particle surface area concentration versus particle size for several different values of the unattached activity fraction, f, are shown in Fig. 5.3. For ^{218}Po,

$$\lambda_A = 3.788 \times 10^{-3} s^{-1}$$

$$S = 8.84 \times 10^{-7}[(1/f) - 1](1 + 7 \times 10^4 r) \text{ nm}^2 \text{ cm}^{-3}.$$

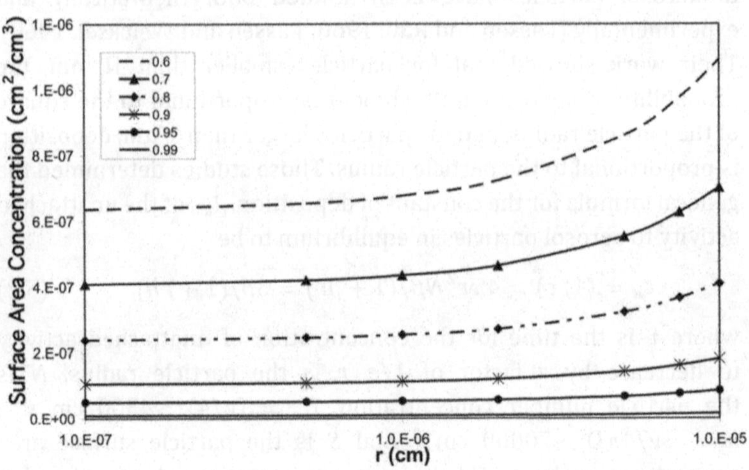

Figure 5.3 Correlation between aerosol surface area and unattached radium A (^{218}Po).

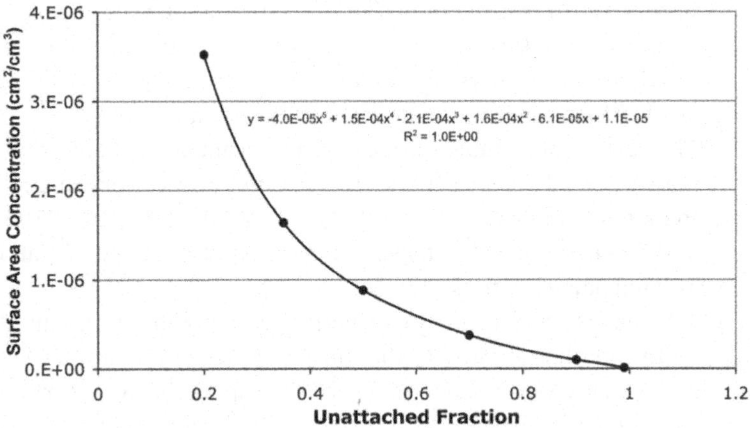

Figure 5.4 Relationship between unattached fraction and particle surface area concentration.

Figure 5.4 suggests that for the same concentration of the unattached activity fraction, the surface area of the particles will not depend on particle size for particles smaller than 10 nm (Ruzer and Apte, 2005). Calibration of this technique should be done with monodispersed spherical particles. Practical measurements of polydispersed and nonspherical particles in the nanometer range will need to be presented in the units of "equivalent surface area," i.e., the surface area of monodispersed particles, which correspond to the same concentration of the unattached fraction.

5.2 Conclusion

1. For a constant value of the unattached fraction, f, the airborne particle surface area is practically independent of particle size in the size range 1–100 nm.
2. The measurement of airborne particle surface area by this method is practical for polydisperse nanoparticles.
3. This method will not be sensitive to the very small nanoparticles, because their contribution to the total surface area is small because surface area is proportional to the diameter squared.

4. According to calculations (Eq. (5.5)), the measurement of unattached ^{214}Bi ($\lambda_c = 5.864 \times 10^{-4}$ s^{-1}) for the same f provides an opportunity to measure surface area that are smaller than those for unattached ^{218}Po by a factor of 8.
5. The lowest detectable surface area concentration is approximately 2×10^{-7} cm^{-1}, or 2×107 nm^2 cm^{-3}, which corresponds to number concentrations of 2×10^6, 7×10^4, 1.8×10^4, 2700, and 70 cm^{-3} for monodispersed aerosols of 2, 10, 20, 50, and 100 nm particles, respectively.
6. The highest surface area concentration that can be measured by this method is close to that measured when the unattached activity fraction is close to 0.05 (corresponding to a surface area of 1.5×10^{-5} cm^{-1} = 1.5×10^9 nm^2 cm^{-3}. For an aerosol of 100 nm monodispersed particles, this corresponds to approximately 50,000 particles per cm^3.

References

Banse DF, et al. (2001) *J Aerosol Sci* **32**, 157–161.

Butterweck G, et al. (2001) *Radiat Prot Dosim* **94**, 247–250.

Croft JF, Perry KEG (1962) An experimental study of the behaviour and detection of hazardous radon releases in air. AEE Winfrith, w. 5356. UK Atomic Energy Authority Reactor Group Report, AEEW – R 149.

Dokukina VL, Ruzer LS (1976) All-Union Institute of Physico-Technical and Radiotechnical Measurements (VNIIFTRI), Moscow, **30**(60) (in Russian).

Donaldson K, Li XY, MacNee W (1998) *J Aerosol Sci* **29**, 553.

Lassen L, Rau G (1960) *Zeitschift f Physik* **160**, 504.

Lassen L, Weicksel, H (1961) *Zeitschift f Physik* **161**, 339–345.

Maynard AD (2003) *Ann Occup Hyg* **47**(2), 123–144.

NSF (2003) NSF Workshop Report on Emerging Issues in Nanoparticle Aerosol Science and Technology, University of California, Los Angeles, June 27–28, 2003.

Oberdörster G, Oberdörster E, Oberdörster J (2005) *Environ Health Perspect* **113**, 823–839.

Ruzer LS (1964) The manner of determination of the absorbed dose upon the inhalation of radon. Patent No. 165250, *Bull Invent* **18**, USSR (in Russian).

Ruzer LS, Apte MG (2005) Radon as a potential experimental tool in aerosol dosimetry. *Frontiers in Aerosol Dosimetry Research*, Irvine, California, October 24–25, 2005.

Ruzer LS, Sextro RG (1997) *Prot Dosimetry* **71**, 135–140.

Wilson WE, Stanek J, Pui DYH, Han HS (2004) Use of the electrical aerosol detector as an indicator for the total particle surface area deposited in the lung. *Symposium on Air Quality Measurement Methods and Technology*, Research Triangle Park, NC.

Chapter 6

Local Deposition of Nanoparticles in the Human Lung

In this chapter, we discuss a method based on existing research using 1 nm particulate radon decay products as an experimental tool in the study of local lung deposition and dosimetry for nanoaerosols. The health effects of aerosols in air pollution are discussed widely in the scientific literature. During the past 10 years, the need to understand the relationships between aerosol exposure and biological effects has become particularly important due to the rapid development of nanotechnology and adoption of nanomaterials by industry. The understanding of the relationship between aerosol concentration in the breathing air and particle deposition in different portions of the lung remains poor, in spite of several decades of research. The method proposed here will allow for better collection of data that can be used to research the impact of local particle deposition on the etiology of health effects. Without direct validation through measurement of aerosol deposition and dose, uncertainty in estimates from inhalation models will persist.

In this chapter, we discuss a proposed method for dose assessment of nanoaerosols, i.e., particles in the range of 1–100 nm. Nanometer aerosols are particles of extremely small sizes. A

Nanoparticles in Humans: Experiments, Methods, and Strategies
Lev S. Ruzer

ISBN 978-981-4463-16-4 (Hardcover), 978-981-4463-17-1 (eBook)
www.panstanford.com

radioactive marker for these particles must be even smaller in size in order not to distort experimental results. We propose as an experimental tool the smallest radioactive nanoparticle, 1 nm, called unattached activity of radon progeny. These particles form naturally by radioactive decay of the inert radioactive gas radon.

The goal in these human experiments is to measure the local lung deposition of nanoaerosols by measurement of the gamma-activity of radon progeny. After inhalation of the mixture of monodispersed aerosols in the nanometer range, labeled with 1 nm unattached activity of radon progeny, which build up naturally due to radioactive decay of inert radioactive gas radon, the distribution of the gamma-activity in the lung is measured.

Because each locally deposited nanoparticle is associated with measured gamma-quantum or gamma-activity, the gamma-activity itself quantitatively represents locally deposited nanoparticles, i.e., local nanoparticle dose. After inhalation, the gamma-activity distribution in the lung represents local distribution of nanoparticles, since these particles are radiolabeled with radon progeny. Measurements are conducted after exposure. Because the goal is to assess dose to the lung directly, data on measured exhaled fraction of aerosols is not needed.

There are many gaps in our knowledge of aerosol deposition in the respiratory system. Although many of these gaps are particle size independent, improved methods for assessing the deposition of particles in the nanometer range need to be developed in order to improve risk assessment and dosimetry of nanoaerosols (NIOSH, 2005). Specific gaps include

- regional dosimetry of nanomaterials;
- measurement studies of nanoparticle surface area in the workplace.

Due to the very large ratio of surface area to number for nanoparticle aerosols, the relationship between particle deposition and surface area of deposited particles becomes crucial at the nanoscale. Thus, the particle surface area and number dosimetry must be addressed simultaneously.

The items in the above list may be divided into those that represent gaps in environmental measurement techniques and those that represent gaps in human exposure assessment and dosimetric methods for these aerosols.

Here, we discuss a new approach to the measurement of aerosol surface area concentration based on the rate of deposition of the unattached activity of radon progeny on aerosol particles.

One experimental approach that addresses exposure and dosimetric gaps uses safe doses of radioactive tracer particles. After airborne particles are inhaled, their spatial distribution in the lung can be determined through two- and possibly three-dimensional spectrometric imaging. In recent years, published literature on the risks associated with using radioactive markers in human imaging has matured to the point where reliable and safe protocols have been devised for their measurement.

As mentioned by Oberdörster and colleagues (Oberdörster et al., 2005), it is not clear if there are significant human exposures to airborne-engineered carbon nanotubes or C_{60} fullerene particles. This is of concern, because, for example, at the very low mass concentration of 10 $\mu g/m^3$ of unit density 20 nm particles, the number concentration is greater than 10^6 particles/cm^3. At this concentration, what is the particle surface dose delivered per cm^2 to different lung tissue? Animal studies using ultrafine and nanometer-sized aerosols showed that such particles induced significant pulmonary inflammatory responses as well as effects in extra pulmonary organs (Oberdörster et al., 2005).

Yet, without direct measurements of response in humans with accurate dosimetry we cannot make conclusive estimates of the risks. Examples of the safe use of radioisotopes to label aerosol particles for human inhalation studies are presented in the literature (Philipson et al., 1996; Brown et al., 2000; Kim et al., 2000; Svartengren et al., 2005).

6.1 Safety of Radioactive Markers in Aerosol Exposure Studies

Human studies of exposure to radon progeny can be used to inform an assessment of the safety of its use for measurement of deposition and dosimetry of nanoparticles. If radiation exposure to a radioactive marker is negligible relative to subject's background exposure, it may be assumed that the increased risk to the subject is negligible relative to the background exposures of subjects. The following are three documented settings of exposure to radon and its progeny:

1. Exposure in a general population with average background radon concentration of 20–80 Bq/m^3 and life time exposure duration of 600,000 h (70 years);
2. Exposure of miners, with the permissible concentration 1100 Bq/m^3; and exposure duration of 60,000 h (30 work-years, Ruzer et al., 1995, 2004);
3. The human experiment at the Paul Scherer Institute (PSI), Switzerland (Butterweck et al., 2001); of 20,000 Bq/m^3 and duration of exposure 0.5 h.

A comparison of these three cases shows that radiation exposure in human experiment was less than 1/1000 the magnitude of the life-time background exposure. From a radiation exposure point of view, the experiment in PSI, Switzerland, was safe.

6.2 Assessment of Particle Deposition in Lungs

Until now, experimental data on nanoaerosol deposition in human lungs, especially with regional specificity, have not been available. For larger-size aerosols, mostly bulk deposition data are available based on the difference in concentration in exhaled and inhaled air. However, it is well known that true exposure and biological effect depend on local deposition.

In Ruzer (1970), a correlation was shown between the alpha-dose and gamma-activity of radon progeny measured directly from the lung. This was first studied on animals and then in model experiments. Finally, hundreds of miners in the former Soviet Republics of Tadjikistan, Uzbekistan, and Kazakhstan were studied, and correlation was verified in humans. It was shown that gamma-activity of radon progeny in the lung could be measured using a special vest with strategic placement of NaI(Tl) crystal detectors and standard lead shielding around the thorax of the miners.

The approach of direct measurement of radon progeny may also be used for the assessment of deposition of non-radioactive aerosols, particularly nanometer aerosols, in the lung.

Through radioactive decay, radium produces Rn, which in turn will produce ^{218}Po. Once it is released into the air, about 10–12 molecules of air contents naturally diffuse onto and surround the ^{218}Po atom. These clusters are about 1 nm in diameter and have diffusion coefficient of $\sim$0.06 cm^{2}s^{-1}. They are called unattached activity of radon progeny. Through natural diffusion processes, these Rn progeny are able to deposit on aerosol particles of size ranging from nanometers to micrometers. These clusters possess physical characteristics that can be used in lung dosimetry. The surface to volume ratio of these 1 nm clusters is so large that virtually every molecule contained in them is available at the surface,

Operationally, the concept uses these Po radon progeny as a radiolabel. These particles have a very high diffusion coefficient and readily attach to other particles in the air. When attached, or aggregated with environmental aerosols, these particles are called "attached activity." Given their high diffusion coefficient, their attachment efficiency can approach 100%. Thus almost every particle in the environmental aerosol becomes labeled with a radioactive radon progeny particle, destined to decay and emit gamma particles (^{214}Pb and ^{214}Bi). Particle inhalation experiments may be designed in which relatively low concentration of radon gas is mixed with non-active study aerosol that will subsequently be inhaled by subjects. As the radon atoms decay, their progeny attach to the nonradioactive aerosol particles and radiolabel them.

In this case, every measured gamma-quantum corresponds to a nonradioactive nanometer aerosol particle locally deposited in the lung. So, the measured gamma-radioactivity will represent the dose of non-radioactive nanoaerosols at the target.

The conditions of these experiments will lead to exposures where practically all particles will be attached activity. The concentration of unattached activity will be extremely small because substantial unattached radon progeny concentrations take place only when the aerosol concentration is extremely low. The ratio of attached to unattached activity may be verified during preliminary experimental validations.

The formula for gamma-activity, $A\gamma$, of the attached fraction deposited in the lung is

$$A\gamma = avk(q_b + q_c), \qquad (6.1)$$

where a is a proportional coefficient; v is the volumetric breathing rate; k is the lung deposition coefficient, nondimensional parameter, equal to the ratio of deposited particles to all particles entered the lung; and q_b and q_c are the concentrations of ^{214}Pb and ^{214}Bi, respectively,

After exposure, the local gamma-emission distribution in the lung can be measured using a gamma-spectrometer, with the local activity being proportional to the aerosol deposition (dose). In addition, it may be possible to use the single-photon emission computer tomography (SPECT) scanning to provide a more precise spatial resolution of particle deposition and local dosing (Kao et al., 1997; Piai et al., 2004).

6.3 Previous Experiments with This Method

A study (Ruzer et al., 2004) of more than 250 miners yielded average concentration of (unattached + attached) gamma-radioactive radon decay products (^{214}Pb + ^{214}Bi) of 8.9 (kBq m^{-3}). The average measured activity in the lung was 2.86 kBq. The rugged mining conditions precluded the use of spectrometric instrumentation, so only general activity was measured; however, these experiments demonstrated the feasibility of conducting controlled studies in laboratory conditions where instrumentation is more sensitive and background levels are lower.

In another study (Butterweck et al., 2001) under laboratory conditions, seven nose-breathing and seven mouth-breathing volunteers were exposed to air enriched with unattached radon progeny (3800 Bq m^{-3}). In these measurements, about 10% of the measured activity was due to inhalation of the unattached fraction. In order to optimize these measurements, the researchers used a spectrometric technique with three detectors. The average deposited activity of (^{214}Pb + ^{214}Bi) in the lung was close to 60 Bq. A separate measurement of the activity in the head was also provided.

This experiment may be used to define minimum detection limit for nanoparticle deposition. According to Butterweck et al., the minimum detection limit for gamma-activity in the lung is about 5 Bq (or 5 s^{-1}). According to the formula for radioactive decay (dN/dt), it is possible to calculate the number concentration of unattached fraction in the air using the wire-screen measurement method (previously published in Ruzer and Sextro, 1997). The labeling process of unattached activity to aerosol is published extensively in the literature (see for example Ruzer, 2008). It should be noted that these proposed experiments are different from those described by Butterweck et al. The difference is that they only studied deposition of the unattached activity. We propose to use the unattached activity with the size of 1 nm as a tool to study the lung deposition of particles in nanoparticle range. The particle coagulation process should be at equilibrium in order to accurately measure the particle attachment efficiency of the initially unattached fraction.

6.4 Human Studies

As with all such radiotracer studies, the protocol must meet the approval of an institutional review board (IRB) and radiological scientific review. In these experiments, as in other studies, when radiation is a tool, for example, in using radiolabeled drugs in the study of Alzheimer disease, we have to compare the risk relative to benefit. The use of such experiments will enable us to close the gaps in our knowledge of quantitative assessment of the local deposition of aerosol, and particularly nanoaerosol exposure and risk assessment. So, our goal will be to find the safest possible and most appropriate marker.

The use of unattached activity of radon progeny as a radioactive tracer of deposition in the lung has many advantages:

1. Radon and its progeny belong to the natural background of radioactivity to which the general population is exposed during their lifetime. Therefore, it is easy to assess the additional risks due to their use by the methods proposed.

2. Part of radon progeny, called unattached activity, are 1 nm-sized particles with diffusion coefficient close to 0.06 $cm^2 s^{-1}$ (a size that attaches readily to nanoaerosols), which makes it very attractive as a marker for nanoaerosols with a built-in signal.
3. Radon decay products are easy to generate.
4. Radon decay products are short-lived nuclei.

This is consistent with the use of radiological tracers for other medical research. For human experiments, we propose using a generator of unattached fraction of radon progeny. This could be an environmental chamber such as used in the Swiss research (Butterweck et al., 2001), or using a respirator mask exposure apparatus attached to a small chamber.

6.5 Controlled Protocol for Study of Nanoparticle Lung Deposition in Human Subjects

Controlled experiments where nanometer (or larger) sized aerosols of known diameter are radiolabeled through natural attachment to unattached activity (i.e., becoming attached activity) can be used to trace aerosol lung or surface deposition behavior. To do this, a size-characterized monodisperse aerosol is inserted into an exposure chamber containing particle-filtered air. Rn progeny are also inserted into the chamber at a controlled or known rate. After the nanometer aerosol (labeled with radon progeny) is inhaled into the lungs, the unattached activity with nanometer particles will be locally deposited according to their size depending on some breathing parameters (volume breathing rate, humidity, and temperature).

Many of the experimental parameters for this process will depend upon the exact physical setup of the facility. These physical parameters must be derived experimentally for that facility. Examples of parameters that must be measured are

- The deposition rate at which unattached radon progeny attach to the study aerosol to form attached activity.
- Stability of the concentration of unattached fraction across time and space must be ensured through measurement.

- The stability of deposited particles in the lung will depend on clearance parameters that could vary across individuals.
- The overall sensitivity of the measurements will depend on the instrumentation that is used.

This approach may be used to map aerosol dose to the lung because it can provide graphic information on where and in what amount these particles of different sizes are deposited in the respiratory system.

In order to conduct nanoparticle lung dosimetry, a special facility must be developed. A radon environmental chamber suitable for safe human exposure (Butterweck et al., 2001) should be constructed. A controllable open source of ^{226}Ra should be housed in the chamber. Likewise, a source of the nanoparticles of interest in the deposition experiment should be developed such that it can controllably generate an aerosol in the chamber. For some experiments, these could be monodisperse engineered or natural nanoparticles of different sizes and number concentration (n). In other experiments, the challenge aerosol could be diesel exhaust, tobacco smoke, urban aerosol, or other ultrafine environmental particulate matter of a polydispersed nature.

It will be necessary to develop a phantom calibration procedure with a sealed ^{226}Ra source. The gamma-spectra of this source will be identical to the spectra of radon progeny deposited in the lung, and must have a well-quantified gamma emission rate. The gamma energy emitted from this source will be used to mimic the activity of the radiolabeled aerosol. This calibration is important for generation of a good regional specificity in gamma activity measurements in the lung.

In order to create an accurate mapping of regional deposition of particles in the respiratory system from the gamma emission pattern emerging from the study subject, a soft tissue background image must be created. A number of approaches may be used to do this, but use of magnetic resonance imaging (MRI) may be the most successful. By creating a baseline magnetic resonance image, with the gamma-signal mapped as an overlay, precise regional deposition information can be imaged.

Additionally, a calibrated instrument for measuring the unattached fraction of radon progeny in the chamber is needed (Ruzer and Sextro, 1997). The unattached fraction measurement is needed for the calculation of the attached activity in the chamber and in particle number and surface area doses during an exposure experiment.

The nanoparticle number concentration of the unattached activity can be calculated according to the following formula:

$$N = (1/\lambda_A)A, \qquad (6.2)$$

where N is the unattached activity number concentration (m^{-3}), A the unattached concentration of ^{218}Po ($Bq\ m^{-3}$), and λ_A = ^{218}Po decay constant (s^{-1}).

The surface area concentration in the chamber can be calculated using Eq. 6.2. Calculation of the ratio N/n (where n is the nanoaerosol concentration) in the chamber is a useful parameter, as it describes the attachment ratio of the Rn progeny to the nanoaerosol. For practical purposes, the ratio should remain above 95% for good experimental accuracy.

The next step is to conduct human exposure/dose measurements by placing subjects in the chamber as was done in the Swiss experiments (Butterweck et al., 2001) using a controlled particle source and the radon tracer. First, a set of local gamma-activity deposition experiments in the lung should be conducted using monodisperse nanoparticles to map particle size-dependent deposition regions. This mapping can provide basic information on local deposition as a function of size, but it also serves as a calibration for deposition of polydispersed environmental aerosols. Next the subjects can be exposed in the chamber using the polydispersed nanoaerosols of interest. The duration of exposure in the chamber will depend on the concentration of both the tracer and the nanoaerosol. For guidance, a target activity level should be about $2 \times 10^4\ Bq\ m^{-3}$ and with a duration of about 30 min.

Calculation of the number and surface area dose of monodisperse nanoparticles locally deposited in the lung is done using the gamma-radiation rate measurement such as NaI detector pulse counting, or SPECT scanning, as discussed above. This measured rate is compared against the standard radium source from the phantom measurements also discussed above.

Finally, human measurements of polydisperse nanoaerosol of interest can be made with chamber exposure experiments. The local distribution of the regional dose to the lung can be calculated in units of number and surface area. The measured activity is proportional to the dose of nanoaerosol, with a number of proportionality corrections as described in Ruzer et al. (2004). However, improvements on these proportionalities must come from future research using this method.

6.6 Discussion and Conclusion

Measurement of aerosol deposition and human lung dosimetry is very complicated. First, it is still very difficult to measure the particle size distribution of aerosol particles in the breathing zone of humans. However, even if such data were available, there is a lack of experimental data on local deposition of nanoparticles in human. Therefore, direct measurement of lung deposition parameters is still needed in order to validate the results of modeling and animal studies. We have discussed the potential use of the unattached fraction of radon progeny as a radioactive marker, which can be used as an experimental tool in measurement of local deposition parameters and dosimetry of nanoaerosols.

Although many of the measurement components of this proposed method are well established, it will be necessary to conduct a study to develop and refine a protocol that successfully integrates the parts into a method that meets the objectives of improved nanoparticle dosimetry.

Before implementing the method, some key activities need to be performed:

1. Study of the applicability of this method for particles smaller than 10 nm;
2. Sensitivity of the measurements as a function of instrument used;
3. Developing a phantom calibration procedure, including the use of a known source of gamma-radioactivity;

4. Study of the stability of the unattached progeny over time and space;
5. Experimental determination of physical parameters for the exposure facility.

Review of literature on environmental health in the new rapidly developing nanotechnology industry shows that the problem of exposure has not been adequately assessed (Oberdörster, 2005). Workers' health and safety are of initial concern, as occupational groups are likely to be among the first to be exposed to elevated concentrations of nanomaterials. A gap exists between the existing particle measurement methods and those truly appropriate for nanoaerosol exposure assessment. Until now, the primary tools available for the measurement of nano-sized aerosols have been condensation particle counters (CPCs) and different mobility analyzers (DMAs). However, both methods suffer mainly due to the low probability with which in this range of sizes nanoparticles are charged (NSF, 2003).

A new instrument on the market, the nanoparticle surface area monitor (TSI 3550, Nanoparticle Surface Area Monitor, 2005), is used for the assessment of deposited surface area (DSA) in the lung. Lung deposition estimates from this instrument are based on correlation developed (Wilson et al., 2004) between the electrical signal and modeled DSA. The instrument is said to be capable of detecting particles with diameter down to 10 nm. Another attempt to solve the problem of surface area assessment, previously presented in Maynard (2003), is based on simultaneous number and mass concentration measurements.

Even with improved aerosol instrumentation for nanoparticles, the issue of respiratory tract deposition quantization cannot be resolved without a direct localized measurement of particle dose.

The Swiss experiments discussed above and the measurements of miners as a model for experiments that can be performed in laboratory conditions can provide accurate data on human breathing characteristics, deposition, lung dosimetry, and the assessment of true effectiveness of respirators.

Clearly, all human experiments with nanometer particles labeled with radioactive markers need careful consideration from the point of view of both radioactive and non-radioactive nanometer aerosols safety. Still, in the balance, the scientific need for information from good human lung dosimetry experiments suggests that the problem should be considered.

Interspecies variability in respiratory system morphology and physiology is so great that similar data will be impossible to obtain in animal experiments.

From these observations, the following conclusions can be made:

1. Unattached activity of radon progeny (as a radioactive marker) can be used in a controlled manner that provides minimal risk in human studies under laboratory conditions.
2. Particle deposition, lung dosimetry, measurement of the breathing characteristics for nanometer-sized particles may be measured by noninvasive techniques under laboratory conditions, in the range of exposures described in this chapter.

References

Brown JS, Kim CS, Reist PC, Zeman KL, Bennett WD (2000) Generation of radiolabeled "soot-like" ultrafine aerosols suitable for use in human inhalation studies. *Aerosol Sci Technol* **32**, 325–337.

Butterweck G, et al. (2001) *Radiation Prot Dosimetry* **94**(3), 247–250 (2001).

Kao CH, Chang Lai SP, Shen YY, Lee JK, Wang SJ (1997) Technetium-99m tetrofosmin SPECT imaging of lung masses: A negative study. *J Nucl Med* **38**, 1015–1019.

Kim CS, Jaques PA (2000) Respiratory dose of inhaled ultrafine particles in healthy adults. *Philos Trans R Soc Lond* **358**, 2693–2705.

Maynard AD (2003) Estimating aerosol surface area from number and mass concentration measurements. *Ann Occup Hyg* **47**(2), 123–144.

National Science Foundation (2003) NSF Workshop Report on Emerging Issues in Nanoparticle Aerosol Science and Technology (NAST). University of California, Los Angeles, California.

NIOSH (2005) Strategic plan for NIOSH nanotechnology research: Filling the knowledge gaps. Nanotechnology Research Program, National Institute for Occupational Safety and Health, Centers for Disease Control and Prevention. Draft.

Oberdörster G, Oberdörster E, Oberdörster J (2005) *Environ Health Perspect* **113**, 823–839.

Philipson K, Falk R, Gustafson J, Camner P (1996) Long-term clearance of ^{195}Au-labelled Teflon particles in humans. *Exp Lung Res* **22**, 65–83.

Piai DB, Quagliatto R, Toro I, Neto C, Etchbehere E, Camargo E (2004) The use of SPECT in preoperative assessment of patients with lung cancer. *Eur Respir J* **24**, 258–262.

Ruzer LS (1970) Doctor's Dissertation. VNIIFTRI, Moscow, USSR.

Ruzer LS (2008) Assessment of nanoparticles surface area by measuring of unattached fraction of radon progeny. *J Nanopart Res* **10**, 761–766.

Ruzer LS, Nero AV, Harley NH (1995) Assessment of lung deposition and breathing rate of underground miners in Tadjikistan. *Radiation Prot Dosimetry* **58**, 261–265.

Ruzer LS, Harley NH (2004) *Aerosol Handbook: Measurement, Dosimetry, and Health Effects*, CRC Press, New York.

Ruzer LS, Sextro RG (1997) Assessment of very low aerosol concentrations by measuring the unattached fraction of ^{218}Po. *Prot Dosimetry,* **71**, 135–140.

Svartengren M, Wiebert P, Sanchez-Crespo A, Seitz J, Falk R, Philipson K, Kreyling WG, Sommerer K, Larson S (2005) Retention of ultrafine 35 and 100 nm carbonaceous particles in healthy and affected human lungs. In: *Proceedings of Frontiers in Aerosol Dosimetry Research*, October 24–25, 2005, Irvine, California.

Wilson WE, Stanek J, Pui DYH, Han HS (2004) Use of the electrical aerosol detector as an indicator for the total particle surface area deposited in the lung. *Symposium on Air Quality Measurement Methods and Technology*, Research Triangle Park, NC.

Chapter 7

Exposure and Dose in Nanoaerosols Studies

The nanotechnology industry is rapidly growing with promises of substantial benefits that will have significant global economic and scientific impacts applicable to a whole host of areas from engineering and electronics to environmental remediation and medical healthcare. However, at present, there is growing concern over the safety of nanomaterials with respect to occupational, consumer and environmental exposures and associated health effect.

Particularly, information on nanomaterial exposure, dosimetry, risk assessment, and health effect is negligible.

According to Kulinowski et al., "There's a lot more data now than there was back in the early days. Between 2001 and 2008 (the last year for which complete data are available), the annual NanoEHS publication rate grew between 20–120% per year with over 3600 individual papers." Unfortunately, however, "it becomes equally difficult to say that all these data are conclusive. A recent analysis found that much of the 'nanotoxicology' research is done in vitro, focusing on acute toxicity and mortality induced by native nanoparticles, with limited relevance to human health."

Nanoparticles in Humans: Experiments, Methods, and Strategies
Lev S. Ruzer

ISBN 978-981-4463-16-4 (Hardcover), 978-981-4463-17-1 (eBook)
www.panstanford.com

Up to present time, available quantitative data related to dosimetry of nanomaterials, and particularly aerosolized nanoparticles are very difficult to find.

As Geraci discusses in NIOSH (2009), in terms of nanoparticles we still do not know the nature and extent of hazard, exposure, and risk; what measure to use; limitations of controls and protection; and appropriate limits. There are no specific exposure limits.

According to The Friends of the Earth Nanotechnology Project (2009), there is

> no consistent nomenclature, terminology and measurement standards to characterize and describe nanoparticles and exposure. Inadequate understanding of nanotoxicity, in particular to determine whether acceptable exposure limits exist. No effective methods to measure and assess workplace exposure to nanoparticles; no data on existing or predicted workplace exposure.
>
> Despite the hundreds of products containing nanomaterials that are already being manufactured commercially, and the emerging body of scientific literature demonstrating the serious risk associated with nanotoxicity, there are still no laws to manage workplace exposure and to ensure workers' safety. This suggests that governments have learnt little from their experiences with asbestos.

The health effects from aerosols in air pollution are discussed widely in the scientific literature. During the past 10 years, the need to understand the relationships between aerosol exposure and biological effects has become especially important due to rapid development of a new, revolutionary industry—nanotechnology.

The understanding of the relationship between aerosol concentration in the breathing air and particle deposition in different portions of the lung remains poor, in spite of several decades of research. There are many gaps in our knowledge of aerosols in the nanometer range, which need to be filled in order to improve risk assessment and dosimetry of nanoaerosols, including:

1. nanoparticle dosimetry and risk assessment;
2. evaluation of pulmonary deposition and translocation of inhaled nanomaterials;

3. lack in the systematic approach for the assessment of the main cause of the health effect—nanoaerosol dose;
4. measurement studies of nanoparticle surface area concentrations in the workplace.

Some of the gaps are substantial for aerosols in all ranges of sizes, but majority are especially important for the particles in the range 1–100 nm.

The problem presented in this chapter in the form of nanoaerosol dosimetric road map, where the nanoaerosol dose assessment is divided to particular steps each of it contributing to the main dosimetric goal.

According to the EPA (1996), in epidemiological studies, an index of exposure from personal or stationary monitors of selected pollutants is analyzed for associations with health outcomes, such as morbidity or mortality. However, it is a basic tenet of toxicology that the dose delivered to the target site, not the external exposure, is the proximal cause of a response. Therefore, there is increased emphasis on understanding the exposure–dose–response relationship.

Exposure is what gets measured in the typical study and what gets regulated; dose is the causative factor. The measurement or assessment of the dose in practice, however, presents substantial difficulties, and as a surrogate of the dose the term "exposure" is used.

7.1 Exposure: Definitions

The term "exposure" came to the aerosol field from the study of the effect of gases. Aerosol science, including epidemiological studies of the health effect of aerosol exposure, was developed mainly in the second half of the 20th century. In 1924, German chemist Fritz Haber proposed the following definition of exposure:

> For each war gas, the amount (c) present in one cubic meter of air expressed in milligrams and multiplied by the time (t) in minutes necessary for the experimental animal inhaling this air to obtain a lethal effect. The bigger this product ($c \times t$), the greater is the toxicity of the war gas.

The definition of exposure in the case of aerosols is much more complicated. The main difference in dosimetry between gases and aerosols is that aerosol distribution is spatially and temporally uneven and aerosol deposited in the lungs is non-uniform. The reason for this is that respirable fractions of aerosols consist of particles with diameters ranging from nanometers to 10 μm. Therefore, their airborne particle size distribution and their deposition inside the lungs are very uneven.

According to the National Academy of Science report, the definition of exposure is: "An event that occurs when there is contact at a boundary between humans and the environment with a contaminant of a specific concentration for an interval of time; the units are concentration multiplied by time."

From our point of view, this definition is not free from some contradiction. If exposure is an event, it cannot be expressed in physical units.

A statistical definition of exposure has been proposed in Ott (1966):

> An exposure at some instant of time is a joint occurrence of two events:
>
> 1. the pollutant of concentration C is present at a particular location in space at a particular time, and
> 2. the person is present at the same time and location in space.

A later definition NAS (1991) addresses the notion that the target remains important, and also that different parts of the target can receive different exposures at the same time.

The last definition is more suitable for aerosols, because it takes into account the specific aerosol problem of non-uniformity.

In the *Guidelines of Exposure Assessment*, a slightly different definition was proposed:

> Exposure—Contact of a chemical, physical, or biological agent with outer boundary of an organism. Exposure is quantified as the concentration of the agent in the medium in contact integrated over the time duration of that contact.

In all these definitions, the key word is contact, which means that in the case of aerosols only breathing zone measurement concentration or particle size distribution should be used for the exposure and particle size measurement. If concentration (and particle size characterization) is provided at a distance from the breathing zone, the correlation should be established between breathing zone and sampling site measurement.

The problem with all of these definitions is that it is not clear in which of them the exposure is a physical value or an event. However, it is clear from all exposure definitions that this term should not be used for the substitution of the dose as a cause of the effect.

Ruzer et al. (2004) present the definition of dose in case of aerosols:

> Dose is the specific quantity of aerosols delivered to a target site that is directly responsible for a biological effect.

The term "quantity" is defined as follows:

1. In the case of radioactive aerosols, deposited energy per unit mass for alpha, beta, or gamma radiation is expressed in units of J/kg (Gray) or rads (100 erg/g) or the equivalent.
2. In case of non-radioactive aerosols, quantity is the deposited number of particles, surface area, or mass of a discrete particle size.
3. The term "directly" means that dose is a quantity of the deposited amount of aerosol particles after the completion of all biokinetic processes.

Unfortunately, the term dose is easier to define than measure in practice. Therefore, in many studies the exposure is measured as a concentration multiplied by time, and attempts were made to find correlation between exposure (which is, strictly speaking, only surrogate of the cause of effect – dose) and the health effect. We present two of such studies.

7.2 Examples of Exposure–Effect Study without Dose Assessment

We think it makes sense to analyze these studies especially because we are now at the beginning of the new global problem: assessment of the dose and health effect of nanoparticles. The similarity is that both in this case and in that of radon and its progeny, we have to study two groups of separate problems: dosimetry and health effect. The difference is that in case of radiation in general and problem of radon and its progeny in particular, there were many studies on correlations between radon and its progeny both in terms measurements and health effect, including on human. Unfortunately, similar data for nanoparticles are not available right now.

We illustrate this with results of two studies: BEIR VI and Darby et al. (2004). Remarkably, in BEIR VI, the distribution of radon and its progeny concentrations in mines of 11 different countries were presented and analyzed together with data on lung cancer mortality among miners.

Darby et al. (2004) collected and analyzed similar very important data on radon concentrations in different countries in Europe. Unfortunately, they try to connect radon concentration with lung cancer mortality of the general population despite the fact that only radon progeny, not radon itself, is responsible for the biological effect. So, it is a classic case when not a dose as a cause of the effect but rather dose's surrogate was studied, and the correlation and the real cause were not established. But that is not all.

In this study the authors found that "the absolute risks of lung cancer by age 75 years at usual radon concentrations of 0, 100, and 400 Bq/m^3 would be about 0.4%, 0.5%, and 0.7%, respectively, for lifelong non-smokers, and about 25 times greater (10%, 12%, and 16%) for cigarette smokers."

It is obvious that if we take into account uncertainty in the risk assessment in this case, the numbers 0.4%, 0.5%, 0.7% and 10%,12%, 16% will be the in the range of errors, i.e., the same. By the way, these concentrations are considerably lower than permissible concentrations for mines.

In Table D-12 of BEIR VI results of "average exposures" in "Average Working Levels" (WLM) are presented for 11 countries (China—

286.0, Czechoslovakia—196.8, France—59.4, Canada, USA—578.6, etc.). We know that the uncertainty in the exposure assessment is in the order at least of tens of percents. So, we cannot trust these data with tenths of WLM.

Our study on dosimetry and health effect on miners in Tajikistan (Ruzer et al. 1995) suggested that different groups of miners got substantially different exposure (dose) and different lung cancer mortality. So averaging in this case can lead to additional uncertainty.

It seems that in epidemiological studies, some sort of tendency exists to present as much as possible cases of effect (mortality, morbidity, etc.) in order to get good statistics. With such tendency, old and questionable data on concentrations are often used, even based on data on ventilation. So, our good statistics on mortality in such case are compromised by bad dosimetry.

7.3 Nanoparticle: Definition

In aerosol science, a particle is defined as a small object that behaves as a whole unit in terms of its transport and properties. It is further classified according to size: In terms of diameter, fine particles have a range between 100 and 2500 nm, while ultrafine particles, on the other hand, are sized between 1 and 100 nm.

Like ultrafine particles, nanoparticles are sized between 1 and 100 nanometers, though the size limitation can be restricted to two dimensions.

Nanoparticles may or may not exhibit size-related properties that differ significantly from those observed in non-nanoparticles or bulk material.

There is no accepted international definition of a nanoparticle, but one given in the new PAS71 (the British Standards Institution, BSI) document developed in the UK is: "Particle with one or more dimensions at the nanoscale." Correspondingly, the nanoscale is defined as "having one or more dimensions of order of 100 nm or less." There is a note associated with this definition: "Novel properties that differentiate nanoparticles from the bulk material typically develop at a critical length scale of under 100 nm."

This makes the size of particles or the scale of its features the most important attribute of nanoparticles.

What is different about a nanoparticle?

There is no strict dividing line between nanoparticles and non-nanoparticles. The size at which materials display different properties to the bulk material is material dependant and can certainly be claimed for many materials much larger in size than 100 nm. Most experts in the UK and the USA define nanoparticles as particles smaller than 100 nm. However, in Japan, for example, particles between 50 and 100 nm are classified as "ultrafine" and only those below 50 nm in one dimension as nanoparticles. Even some agencies in the USA use the term "ultrafine" to describe particles under 100 nm (usually in connection with natural or incidental nanoparticles).

The data shown in Fig. 7.1 demonstrate that nanoparticles appeared to be more inflammatory in the lung than microscale particles. However, if the data were plotted against the surface area instead of the mass, response was identical for both nano- and larger particles. In other words, in principle there is no difference between the nanoparticles, fine particles and bulk materials. The difference is that in case of nanoparticles, the ratio of the number of molecules on the surface to all molecules of the particle, "surface to volume ratio" (SVR), is much higher than that of fine particles or bulk materials.

The graph illustrating the portion of molecules on the surface to all molecules of the particle as a function of particle size is shown in Fig. 7.2. It is clear from this graph that for nanoparticles close to 1 nm in diameter, the surface-area-to-volume ratio is close to 1 (100%). In this chapter, we propose the use of radioactive particles with the size of 1 nm in diameter and diffusion coefficient $\sim$0.06 cm^2 s^{-1} as an experimental tool in the study of nanoparticles. It is also clear from the same graph that for spherical particles with diameter of 100 nm, the surface-to-volume ratio will be $\sim$0.03 (3%). So, the range of sizes of nanoparticle in terms of surface-area-to-volume is from 0.03 to 1.0. Based on this consideration, we propose another definition for nanoparticles based on the portion of molecules on the surface in relation to all molecules of the particle. As an appropriate number for this boundary portion, we propose 3% or 0.03, which according to the graph in Fig. 7.2 corresponds to spherical particles with diameter of 100 nm.

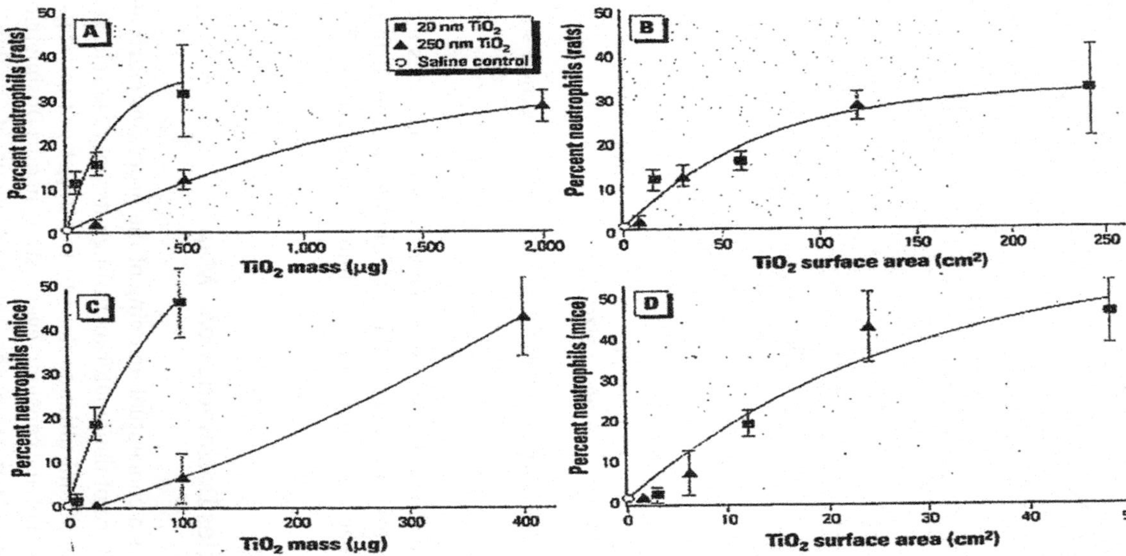

Figure 7.1 Percentage of neutrophils in lung lavage of rats (A, B) and mice (C, D) as indicators of inflammation 24 h after intratracheal instillation of different mass doses of 20 nm and 250 nm TiO_2 particles in rats and mice. (A, C) The steeper dose response of nano-sized TiO_2 is obvious when the dose is expressed as mass. (A, D) The same dose response relationship as in (A, C) but with the dose expressed as the particle surface area; this indicates that the particle surface area seems to be a more appropriate dosimetric for comparing the effects of different-size particles, provided they are of the same chemical structure (anatase TiO_2 in this case). Data show mean ± SD.

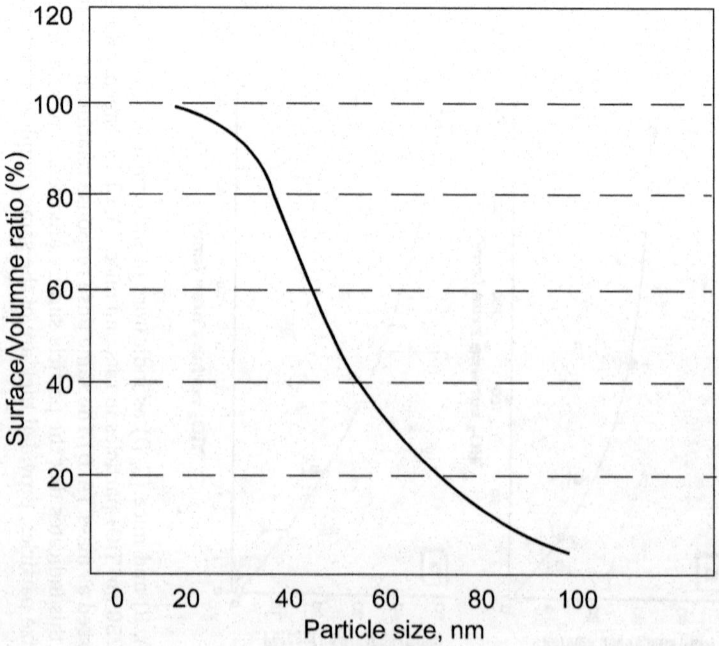

Figure 7.2 Nanoparticle surface-to-volume ratio (%) versus particle size (nanometers).

Our proposed definition of nanoparticles is: "Nanoparticles are particles which have the ratio of number of molecules on the surface to all particle molecules—surface to volume ratio (SVR)—of 3% (0.03) or higher."

7.4 Nanoparticles Dosimetric Road Map

Figure 7.3 presents a conceptual mapping of the processes starting with the manufacture of nanomaterial, through its possible release into the environment and ultimate dose to the target cell in lungs and other organs. Let us consider every step in our Dosimetric Nanoaerosols Road Map from the point of view of available approach, methods and measurement technique. We begin with the left branch, which describes the study of airborne nanoparticles.

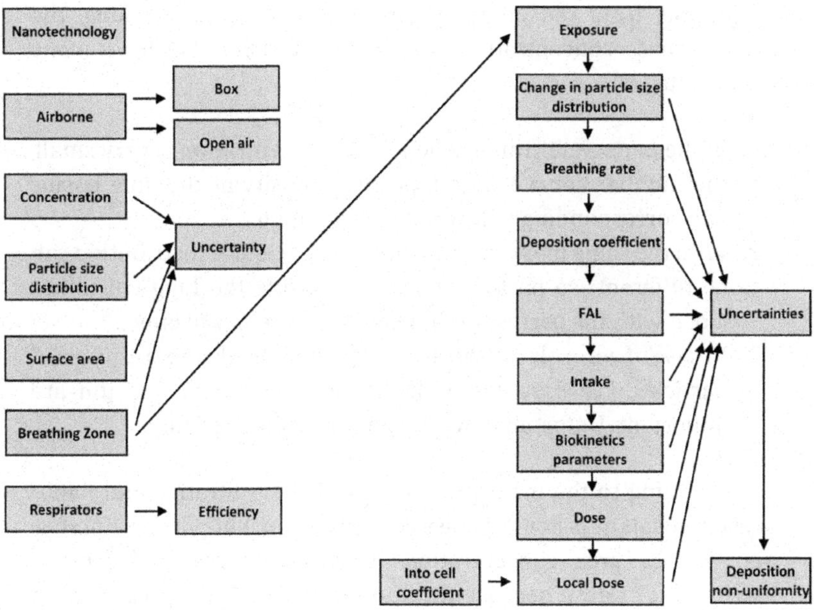

Figure 7.3 Nanoparticles dosimetric road map.

Manufacturing and handling processes for nano-sized materials are widely variable. For example, the materials may be fabricated in a fluidic system closed to the environment (e.g., colloidal suspension of metallic crystals formed in a liquid reaction vessel), or in an open-air system where they may directly mix with ambient air (e.g., manufacture of carbon black using combustion techniques). For each nanotechnology, the potential for fugitive emissions leading to an airborne concentration can be different. Information on the release of the nanomaterial into the air for different nanomaterial manufacturing is very scarce.

It should be noted that the problem of metric in nanoaerosol concentration is complicated. First, nanoaerosols often exist in practice as a structure not as a single particle with the size at least in one dimension in the range from 1 to 100 nm in diameter. So, generally speaking, it is not always possible to use diameter itself as a characteristic of the particle.

Second, from the point of view of the dose to the lung, the aerosol mass concentrations as a characteristic also have many disadvantages:

1. In the nanometer range when mass concentration is very small, the number concentration, particle density at the lung tissue, and correspondingly dose can be very high.
2. With the same mass concentration, particle size distribution can be different; so particle deposition inside the lung will differ along with the corresponding dose and biological effect.
3. In case of aerosols for the dose assessment only the "respirable" particles, i.e., particles with diameter less than 5–7 μm are important. Unfortunately, this limit is itself uncertain.

According to the majority of the studies of ultrafine and nano-sized aerosols, it is not the mass concentration, but particle number and surface area concentrations that should be used for the assessment of dose because they appear to be better predictors of health effects.

In this chapter, we present the new idea on nanoparticle surface area measurement.

7.5 Nanoparticle Surface Area Measurements

Particle surface area is currently considered to be an important toxicological criterion for assessing inhalation exposure. Currently, however, there is a need to develop and expand methods available by which particle surface area concentrations can be assessed in the workplace. The main concern is with free nanoaerosols that are more available for absorption and distribution within the body. Investigators found that when lung burdens and clearance rates were expressed as a function of the surface area, there was a much closer correlation with biological responses.

The special importance of the surface area of nanoparticles in the study of the risk assessment is discussed in Maynard (2003) by comparing the three characteristics: particle number, surface area, and mass concentration.

The use of the particle surface area as a dose metric for nanoaerosols is discussed in many reports: NIOSH (2006), Royal Society (2004), Aitken et al. (2004), SCENIHR (2006), Renn and Roco (2006), and ASCC (2006).

Our proposed approach (Ruzer, 2008) in measuring particle surface area represents a synthesis of:

1. derived direct analytical correlation between the "unattached fraction" of radon progeny and surface area particle concentration in the range of 1–100 nm particle diameter;
2. experimental data on correlation between the unattached fraction of radon progeny and particle surface area for particle diameter in the range of 44 nm to 2.1 μm.

One important property of radon decay products is that after alpha decay of radon, the newly formed atom of ^{218}Po becomes surrounded by a small number of molecules (around 10 to 12). Such molecular clusters, referred to as unattached progeny, with sizes in the range 1–4 nm and diffusion coefficients of approximately 0.06 $cm^2\ s^{-1}$, can be potentially useful as a marker in the studies of properties of non-radioactive aerosols, especially nanoaerosols. These progeny may remain unattached, or may become associated with existing aerosols. It seems reasonable that there should be some correlation between unattached activity and aerosol concentration. It is likely that lower aerosol concentrations will lead to larger fractions of unattached activity. If this relationship can be quantified, then the unattached activity fraction of radon progeny can be used as a measure of airborne particle concentration. This idea was illustrated by an experimental study with spherical polystyrene particles in the size range 0.3–2.1 μm, i.e., outside of the nanometer range. The procedure for measuring the relationship between the unattached activity fraction and particle concentration consists of passing the radon-exposed air through a device with two channels: one with only an open filter and one with a diffusion or wire screen. The measurement of these parameters should be provided by means of an "unattached activity generator," a device capable of generating a regulated unattached activity fraction. Such generators were described in Dokukina and Ruzer (1976) and Butterweck et al. (2001).

7.6 Nanoparticle Respirators' True Effectiveness Measurements

The problem of respirator efficiency has been discussed in many reports (Renn and Roco, 2005). It is well known that the determining factor that governs the effectiveness of respiratory protective equipment (RPE) is not absolute penetration through the filter, but rather face-seal leakage, which bypasses the device.

In Ruzer et al. (1995), the new idea for measuring the true efficiency of respirators was used based on direct measurement of the gamma-activity of radon progeny in lungs of human.

Let us denote the following:

A_0: measured gamma-activity in the lung of miners before entering radon atmosphere; (background measurement);

A_1–A_0: measured gamma-activity in the lung of miners without wearing respirator;

A–A_0: measured gamma-activity in the lung of miners with respirator.

Then respirator effectiveness will be $(A - A_0)/(A_1 - A_0)$ 100%; and penetration coefficient $\{1 - [(A - A_0)/(A_1 - A_0)]\}$100%.

Our measurements in mines demonstrated that true respirator efficiency varies from 67% to 95% depending on individual training, duration, and type of work. At the present time, the data on the true effectiveness of respirators, including the face-leakage problem, are unavailable.

7.7 Local Lung Deposition and Dosimetry for Nanoparticles

There is a lack of systematic studies on nanoparticle lung deposition. One of the most important difficulties in the assessment of the dose as a main cause of the effect from aerosols, particularly in the nanometer range, is the lack of information on local deposition in the human lung. We presented our approach to this fundamental problem in Ruzer and Apte (2010).

Operationally, the concept uses this ^{218}Po radon progeny as a radiolabel. These particles have a very high diffusion coefficient and readily attach to other particles in air. When attached, or aggregated, with the environmental aerosol, these particles are called "attached activity." Given their high diffusion coefficient, their attachment efficiency can approach 100%. Thus, almost every particle in the environmental aerosol becomes labeled with a radioactive radon progeny particle, destined to decay and emit gamma particles (^{214}Pb and ^{214}Bi). Particle inhalation experiments may be designed in which relatively low concentrations of radon gas are mixed with a non-active study aerosol that will subsequently be inhaled by subjects. As the radon atoms decay, their progeny attach to the study aerosol particles and thus radiolabel them.

In this case, every measured gamma-quantum corresponds to a non-radioactive aerosol particle in the nanometer range locally deposited in the lung. So, the measured gamma-activity will represent dose of non-radioactive nanoaerosols at the target.

7.8 Human Experiment Safety Problems

As with all such radiotracer studies, the protocol must meet the approval of an institutional review board (IRB) and radiological screening review. In these experiments, as in other studies, when radiation is used as a tool, for example, in using radio labeled drugs in the study of Alzheimer disease, we have to compare the risk relative to benefit. The use of such experiments will enable us to close the gaps in our knowledge. Quantitative assessment of the local deposition of aerosol is at the core of aerosol, and particularly nanoaerosol exposure and risk assessment. So, our goal will be to find the safest possible and most appropriate marker.

The use of unattached activity of radon progeny as a radioactive tracer of deposition in the lung has many advantages:

1. Radon and its progeny belong to the natural background of radioactivity to which the general population is exposed during their lifetime. Therefore, it is easy to assess the additional risks due to their use by the methods proposed.

2. Part of radon progeny, called unattached activity, are 1 nm particles with diffusion coefficient close to 0.06 cm^2 s^{-1} (a size that attaches readily to nanoaerosols), which makes it very attractive as a marker for nanoaerosols with a built-in signal.
3. Radon decay products are easy to generate.
4. Radon decay products are short-lived nuclei.

This is consistent with the use of radiological tracers for other medical research. For human experiments, we propose using a generator of unattached fraction of radon progeny. This could be an environmental chamber such as used in the Swiss research, or using a respirator mask exposure apparatus attached to a small chamber.

Human studies of exposure to radon progeny can be used to inform an assessment of the safety of its use for measurements of deposition and dosimetry of nanoparticles. If radiation exposure to a radioactive marker is negligible relatively to subjects' background exposures, it may be assumed that the increased risk is negligible relatively to the background exposures of the subjects. The following are three documented settings of exposure to radon and its decay products:

1. exposure in a general population with average background radon concentration of 20–80 Bq/m^3; and lifetime exposure duration of 600,000 h (70 years);
2. exposure of miners, with the permissible concentration 1100 Bq/m^3; and exposure duration of 60,000 h (30 work-years);
3. the human exposure experiment in Paul Scherer Institute (PSI), Switzerland, of 20,000 Bq/m^3 and duration of exposure 0.5 h.

A comparison of these three cases shows that radiation exposure in the human experiment was less than 1/1000 the magnitude of the lifetime background exposure. From a radiation exposure point of view the experiment in PSI, Switzerland, was safe.

7.9 Conclusion

In this chapter, we discussed the problem of exposure and dose as a measure and cause of the health effect studies associated with nanoaerosols.

In two studies of the health effect associated with radioactive aerosols presented above, where not the dose itself but rather surrogates of the dose–exposure were used, it was demonstrated that it is impossible to make conclusive assessment of the risk associated with radon and its decay products.

From the different definitions of exposure discussed above, it is clear that some of definitions are not free from contradictions, because in some cases exposure is considered as a physical value in units of concentration multiplied by time, and in others as an event.

It is very important that exposure cannot be considered as a cause of the effect and strictly speaking cannot be used as a substitute of the dose. Of course, we understand that in practice the measurement of the exposure is more simple and cheaper than the dose assessment. We proposed in this chapter a new definition for nanoparticles based on the ratio of molecules on the surface of particle to all molecules (surface-to-volume ratio, S/V).

We suggest that in the study of the health effect associated with nanoparticles, we have to assess the dose, not exposure, as a measure of the effect.

Therefore we propose the Nanoparticles Dosimetric Road Map, consisting of two main branches: assessment of the airborne nanoparticles and assessment of local deposition of nanoparticles in the lung. The Nanoparticles Dosimetric Road Map presents a conceptual mapping of the processes starting with the manufacture of nanomaterial, through its possible release into the environment and ultimately to the dose to the target cell in lungs and other organs.

We presented a new idea for measuring the surface area of nanoparticle by using 1 nm radioactive marker unattached fraction of radon progeny. The same tool was proposed for the safe assessment of the local deposition of nanoparticles in the lungs of humans and the measurement of the true effectiveness of respirators for nanoparticles in laboratory conditions.

References

Aitken RJ, Creely KS, Tran CL (2004) Nanoparticles: An occupational hygiene review. Prepared by the Institute of Occupational Medicine for Health and Safety Executive, Edinburgh. Research Report 174.

ASCC (2006) A review of the potential occupational health and safety implications of nanotechnology. Australian Government, Australian Safety and Compensation Council. http://www.ascc.gov.au/ascc/AboutUs/Publications/ResearchReports/ (accessed on July 1, 2009).

Butterweck G, et al. (2001) *Radiation Prot Dosimetry* **94**(3), 247–250.

Darby S, Hill D, Auvinen A, BarrosDios JM, Baysson H, et al. (2004) Radon in homes and risk of lung cancer: Collaborative analysis of individual data from 13 European case-control studies. *BMJ* **330**, 223.

Dokukina VL, Ruzer LS (1976) All-Union Institute of Physico-Technical and Radiotechnical Measurements (VNIIFTRI), Moscow, **30**(60) (in Russian).

EPA (1996) Review of the National Ambient Air Quality Standards for particulate matter: Policy assessment of scientific and technical information, OAQPS Staff Paper, EPA/452/R-96-013, Office of Air Quality Planning and Standards, Research Triangle Park, NC.

Friends of the Earth Nanotechnology Project (2009) AzoNano.com; Workplace exposure to nanomaterials and the question of will nano be the next asbestos.

Kulinowski K, Director, international council on Nanotechnology; Executive Director, Center for Biological and Environmental Nanotechnology. Temptation, temptation: Why easy answers about nanomaterial risk are probably wrong. http://www.azonano.com/article.aspx?ArticleID=2448.

Maynard AD (2003) Estimating aerosol surface area from number and mass concentration measurements. *Ann Occup Hyg* **47**(2), 123–144.

NIOSH (2006) Current Ultrafine Particle and Nanotechnology-Related Research. National Institute for Occupational Safety and Health, Centers for Disease Control and Prevention October 27, www.cdc.gov/niosh/topics/nanotech/oltrares.html.

Ott WR (1966) Concepts of human exposure to air pollution, *Environ Int* **7**, 179–196.

Renn O, Roco M (2005) Nanotechnology, white paper on nanotechnology (IRGC), Switzerland, Geneva, Shaffer.

Renn O, Roco M (2006) White Paper No. 2, Nanotechnology Risk Governance, With annexes by Roco M, Litten E. IRGC, Geneva, http://www.irgc.org/ Nanotechnology.html.

Royal Society (2004) *Nanoscience and Nanotechnologies*. The Royal Society & The Royal Academy of Engineering. London, UK. July. pp. 36–41.

Ruzer LS, Apte MG (2010) Unattached radon progeny as an experimental tool for dosimetry of nanoaerosols: Proposed method and research strategy, *Inhalation Toxicol* **22**(9), 760–766.

Ruzer LS, Nero AV, Harley NH (1995) Assessment of lung deposition and breathing rate of underground miners in Tadjikistan. *Radiation Prot Dosimetry* **58**, 261–265.

SCENIHR (2006) The appropriateness of existing methodologies to assess the potential risks associated with engineered and adventitious products of nanotechnologies. Health and Consumer Protection Directorate—General, Scientific Committee on Emerging and Newly Identified Health Risks (SCENIHR). Brussels: European Commission. 002/005. http://ec.eiropa.eu/health/ph_risk/documents/synth_report.pdf.

Index